THE
ÁLZHEIMER'S
ANSWERBOOK™

Professional Answers to More Than **250** Questions about Alzheimer's and Dementia

CHARLES ATKINS, MD

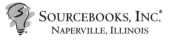

SOURCEBOOKS, INC.®
NAPERVILLE, ILLINOIS

Published by Sourcebooks, Inc.
P.O. Box 4410, Naperville, Illinois 60567-4410
(630) 961-3900
Fax: (630) 961-2168
www.sourcebooks.com

Library of Congress Cataloging-in-Publication Data

Atkins, Charles.
  The Alzheimer's and dementia answer book : professional answers to more than 250 questions about Alzheimer's and dementia / by Charles Atkins.
       p. cm.
  Includes bibliographical references and index.
  1. Alzheimer's disease—Popular works. 2. Senile dementia—Popular works. I. Title.
  RC523.A848 2008
  616.8'31—dc22
                              2008018085

Printed and bound in the United States of America.
       UGI 10 9 8 7 6 5 4 3 2 1

To Ida Marks

Contents

Acknowledgments

First, I need to acknowledge the many families I've met over the years—both in my personal life and in my role as a psychiatrist—who are dealing with a dementing illness. It is from them that I got the inspiration for writing this book, and it is for them that I am writing it.

I'd like to thank the many people who've helped me with this book; their experience, expertise, and time are greatly appreciated: Blanche Agostinelli, APRN; Sigrid Wiemers, APRN; Dianne Davis, APRN; Rajesh Tampi, MD; Albert Zuckerman; Shana Drehs; Doreen Elnitsky, RN; Harvey and Cynthia Atkins; Margaret Munro; Judith Hoberman; Lea Nordicht-Shedd; Gary S. Jayson; Judith Stein; Linda Shaffer; Tracey Violette, OTR/L; Bridget Gallant, LPC; Lisa Hoffman; Vallrie Freeman, MSW; Thomas Reinhardt, MD; Jeannette Mitrukiewitz, LCSW; and MaryAnn Berube, RN.

I'm indebted to the superb medical librarians at Waterbury Hospital Health Center, Linda Spadaccini and Kandace Yuen, for pulling hundreds of articles and scanning the Internet for new sources of information. I'd also like to thank my colleagues at the Department of Behavioral Health of Waterbury Hospital and the staff and administration of Yale's Dorothy Alder Geriatric Assessment Center.

Introduction

I think it's impossible to write a book about Alzheimer's disease and other dementing illnesses without having it become personal. Like many, or even most, Americans, my life has been touched by losing someone I loved through dementia. For me it was my grandmother, who was sharp as a tack through her mid-eighties and then began to lose her memory and other abilities, likely through a series of strokes. I watched as my mother and aunt became caregivers and took on ever greater responsibilities as my grandmother's condition deteriorated. Other family members pitched in expertise and assistance for the necessary financial planning, legal advice, help with moves—from her own apartment, to assisted living, to a nursing home—and emotional support. In the end, my grandmother couldn't recognize her children and required total care.

As my own family was going through this, I was working as a geriatric psychiatrist helping other families plan and strategize. As a young doctor I was impressed by how different each family's treatment of Alzheimer's and other dementias was. While the diagnoses are relatively easy to make, what comes after them, and the layers of planning and information that families and caregivers need, is enormous. This is why I wanted to write this book—when I meet with families in which the mother/father/husband/wife has been diagnosed with a dementia, what strikes me are the barrage of questions they need answered. *"How do you know it's Alzheimer's? How do we handle it when she wanders? How does someone qualify for Medicaid? How do I pick a Medicare D policy for Mom? I read in the paper that substance X is a magic cure, is that true?"*

I've arranged the following material into brief chapters that will hopefully get you to the information you want as quickly as possible. The book can be read straight through, but it's also fine to jump to your particular questions. At the end I've included appendices with contact information for important agencies on aging in your state, as well as advocates for people living in extended-care facilities. There's also, courtesy of Yale University's Dorothy Adler Geriatric Assessment Center, a comprehensive questionnaire that can be of great assistance when you go to seek professional help.

Whether you are a caregiver or a person with a dementing illness, I hope this book eases your journey. Remember that you are not alone; there are millions of other families going through something quite similar. There is help to be had and there is, most certainly, hope.

Chapter 1

WHAT ARE ALZHEIMER'S AND DEMENTIA?

- What is dementia?
- How many people have dementia?
- Is all dementia Alzheimer's disease?
- Is dementia the same thing as senility?
- Isn't dementia just a normal part of getting old?
- Who takes care of people with Alzheimer's and dementia?
- Are Alzheimer's and dementia new diseases?
- Is there more dementia and Alzheimer's now than there used to be?
- Is the rate of dementia higher in the United States than in other countries?
- What are the symptoms of dementia?
- Is memory loss always the first sign of dementia?

What is dementia?

Carl Grant was a partner in a high-powered Manhattan law firm. Two years short of retirement, he found himself struggling with tasks that had once seemed simple. He'd read and then have to reread briefs, at times staring off into space and forgetting what he was doing. He became short-tempered with his secretary, and even accused her of having lost important documents that were later found on his desk, or misfiled in his drawers. In meetings he grew frustrated, needing people to repeat what they'd just said, and having trouble finding the right words.

Where he used to work late hours, he was now frightened of having to drive home after dark, having taken the wrong exit off the highway on multiple occasions. At home, he no longer wanted to get together with friends for bridge. He told his wife Jeanne, "I'm too tired." The truth was that he couldn't keep the cards straight and was afraid that the others would notice. He found himself feeling depressed and thinking that something must be physically wrong. Behind his back his partners grew concerned, and finally confronted Carl and insisted he have a medical evaluation.

Two years later, with his wife, daughter, and son at his side, Carl attended his retirement party, even though he had not come into the office for the past year, after having been diagnosed with early dementia. He smiled and shook hands, although he could not recall the names of most of his colleagues, including his secretary who had been with him for thirty years. He no longer drove, even though he'd often look through the house for his keys. He now spent much of his day in front of the television set, or else would follow his wife around the house, never letting her out of his sight.

Jeanne Grant, a school teacher, made the decision five years before her own scheduled retirement to quit her job and care for Carl at home. As the years passed, it was as though she was watching him move backward in time. She deeply mourned the loss of her husband's quick wit, their physical intimacy, and the travel and social plans the two of them had made for their retirement. At times he could no longer remember her name, and had started to call her "mother." While she often felt burdened, there were still times with Carl where she enjoyed his close-ness, his smile, and memories of their prior life. When Carl became unsteady on his feet, she had the downstairs dining room turned into a bedroom and arranged for aides to help with bathing and getting him to adult day care five days a week.

In his final years, she worried about their combined savings holding out, but made the decision to have live-in care, as Carl now required total assistance at meal times and in the bathroom. He spoke little and became easily upset. In the winter Carl developed pneumonia, and with her children's and physician's input she made the decision to not have Carl hospitalized. He died in his own home three weeks later.

Dementia is a broad term that refers to loss of the brain's ability to function in multiple ways in a person who is otherwise awake and alert. It usually includes memory loss, especially for events that have just happened (short-term memory). Dementias range from mild to totally disabling and in most cases they are progressive—they get worse over time. Dementia affects a person's ability to use language (speak, listen, write, read) and complete tasks; it also affects their behavior and emotions. In the final stages of a progressive dementing illness, people are bedridden, they no longer recognize or remember their loved ones, and they cannot perform the most basic functions to care for themselves. There are over a hundred reported causes of dementia, of which Alzheimer's disease is the most common.

How many people have dementia?

In the year 2000, it was estimated that there were 4.5 million Americans living with Alzheimer's. When we factor in all forms of dementia, this number goes up to more than 6 million. As our population ages, unless a cure or improved treatments are discovered, this number is expected to increase dramatically—almost threefold—by the year 2050.

Other developed countries that have studied their rates of dementia have similar findings.

Is all dementia Alzheimer's disease?

No—but Alzheimer's disease, a brain disease caused by destruction of brain cells (neurons), accounts for between 50–75 percent of cases of dementia. This is followed by vascular dementias, including multi-infarct dementia, which is a result of brain damage caused by multiple small strokes, blocked blood vessels in the brain, or through other processes by which the brain does not receive enough blood and oxygen. Other common causes of dementia include Lewy body disease, dementia caused by chronic alcoholism, HIV/AIDS-related dementia, dementia from head trauma, fronto-temporal dementia (refers to parts of the brain most affected), and the dementia that affects roughly 25–50 percent of people who have Parkinson's disease.

Less common causes of dementia are many, and speak to the numerous ways our brains can be damaged, and include dementia as a result of brain tumors and various infections, including one that results from eating meat infected with "mad cow" disease.

Is dementia the same thing as senility?

Yes, the terms dementia and senility both describe the memory loss and behavioral and emotional changes seen in those affected. Over the years different terms have been used to describe the mental decline seen in Alzheimer's disease and other dementias, including senility, senile dementia, organic brain syndrome, and hardening of the arteries. While Alzheimer's disease is a particular cause of dementia, it is sometimes used to refer to all dementia.

Isn't dementia just a normal part of getting old?

There is a myth that Alzheimer's and dementia are a normal part of aging; they're not. These are diseases of the brain that involve damage and cell loss.

If dementia was a normal part of aging we would expect everyone who lived beyond a certain age to develop it, and this is not the case. It's normal for people to retain their mental abilities into their eighties, nineties, and beyond. Even so, a certain amount of forgetfulness and "senior moments" occur normally with increased age and do not necessarily mean the person has dementia.

Who takes care of people with Alzheimer's and dementia?

Approximately two-thirds of people with dementia are cared for by family and/or friends. This type of in-home care is often referred to as informal or unpaid care. The other third are being cared for in institutional settings—nursing homes, convalescent homes, rest homes, and extended-care facilities.

Women are more often the caregivers for people with dementia by a rate of about two to one. Caregivers are typically spouses/significant others, children, daughters- and sons-in-law, other relatives, and friends.

The majority of informal caregivers provide at least twenty hours a week of unpaid care and over 70 percent live in the same home as the person they are looking after. As the dementia progresses and people require more supervision and hands-on care, the amount of time involved in the caregiving role can increase dramatically.

Are Alzheimer's and dementia new diseases?

No. Dementing illnesses have been a part of the human condition since the beginning of time. References to dementing illnesses go back over two thousand years. Pythagoras, the seventh-century B.C. Greek physician, specifically referred to a process of mental decline in later years where the person returns to an infant-like state. Throughout the Greek and Roman empires, numerous philosophers and physicians (Hippocrates, Plato, Galen, Aristotle, etc.) also commented on and described dementia and loss of mental functioning in later life.

The term "dementia" was first used in the 1700s and is attributed to Phillippe Pinel. Alzheimer's disease was named in the early part of the twentieth century for the physician/scientist, Alois Alzheimer, who identified the tell-tale lesions in the brain (neural plaques and tangles) of people with this disease.

Is there more dementia and Alzheimer's now than there used to be?

Because most dementias occur in later life, it's a fact that the number of people who have dementia is increasing as we live longer. Roughly five million Americans have Alzheimer's disease, and it is estimated that this number will nearly triple by the year 2050.

Is the rate of dementia higher in the United States than in other countries?

In developed countries who have surveyed dementia it appears that the United States, Europe, Japan, Korea, China, Russia, and Canada have similar rates. However, there appear to be subtle differences in the kinds of dementia developed. The U.S. has a higher rate of Alzheimer's disease; and Japan and Russia report higher rates of vascular dementia/multi-infarct dementia.

There is significant inconsistency in how data has been gathered in different countries, especially in the third world, so this question cannot be fully answered. One good source of information on this topic is the World Health Organization's website: www.who.int.

What are the symptoms of dementia?

The easiest way to get a handle on the vast range of symptoms that can be part of a dementia is to break them down into three large categories.

1. Changes in a person's ability to think and to use information (cognition). Specific symptoms in this category include: loss of memory, concentration and focus, the ability to speak and to comprehend language, mathematical capabilities, and reasoning. A person may no longer recognize objects or once-familiar people. Or they may not remember how a particular person is connected to them: *"Our son John was on the phone and he asked, 'who's John?'"*

2. Behavioral and emotional changes. Emotional changes can run the gamut from depression and anxiety to psychosis (hallucination and delusions) and mania (excessive amounts of energy with diminished sleep and very rapid speech). Along with the emotional changes come extremes in behavior that may include aggressiveness—at times with physical assaults on caregivers and others—or the person might lose interest in everything, barely move, and need constant prompting to eat or perform even the most simple task. Wandering from the home or a facility is also common. In certain types of dementia, impulsivity or its opposite, trouble initiating action, can also be prominent symptoms.

3. Loss of the ability to perform tasks typically referred to as activities of daily living (ADLs) and instrumental activities of daily living (IADLs). In early dementia, the ability to perform complex tasks such as balancing a checkbook, preparing a complete meal, driving, and accurately managing medications (IADLs) begin to deteriorate. In the later stages of a progressive dementia, basic skills such as eating, bathing, dressing, and eventually even walking (ADLs) will be lost.

Is memory loss always the first sign of dementia?

No, and as we'll see in Chapter Two, dementias often start with mood and behavior symptoms. Initial symptoms could be a sudden change in personality (as is common in fronto-temporal dementia) or problems with finding words (as is seen in a type of dementia called progressive aphasia). The first observable signs of Alzheimer's may appear as depression, anxiety, or a change in personality:

- *"He was always very quiet and polite—a real gentleman—and then he started to swear and wanted me to have sex every night."*
- *"She used to be so well-spoken and now it takes her forever to say just about anything."*
- *"I don't understand what's happened to Mom: Even when it's obvious that she's wrong about something, she insists that she's right."*

If memory loss is the first sign of early dementia, it may go unrecognized—instead of identifying it as short-term memory loss, the person may experience a vague and disturbing sense that something is wrong.

- *"I used to be able to do this so easily, now I just can't seem to figure it out."*
- *"Why can't I catch on as fast as everyone else? I hate all of this new equipment; it's too hard."*

If you suspect your loved one has dementia, it's important to see your doctor immediately so treatment, and other types of important planning discussed in this book, can begin.

Chapter 2

DEMENTIA BASICS

- Why does Dad remember stuff from fifty years ago, but not from today?
- Is short-term memory the same thing as recall?
- Why does Mom remember some things some of the time?
- Why does my mother think her grandson is her son?
- What are instrumental activities of daily living (IADLs)?
- What are activities of daily living (ADLs)?
- What is mild cognitive impairment (MCI)?
- What are the stages of dementia?
- How long can someone live with Alzheimer's?
- What are the risk factors for developing Alzheimer's?
- If I have a parent with Alzheimer's, what are the chances that I will develop it?
- Are there things you can do to prevent getting Alzheimer's?
- Can dementia be cured?
- If I am getting more forgetful, does that mean I'm going to develop Alzheimer's?

Why does Dad remember stuff from fifty years ago, but not from today?

This commonly asked question has to do with how we remember things and how memory is lost in progressive dementias. Things that happened a long time ago (long-term memory) will remain through the early and middle stages of dementia. Someone may remember the name of their first-grade teacher even when they are no longer able to recall where they currently live or the name of their spouse. It can be confusing and frustrating for family members to have a loved one who can still accurately describe the rules of baseball they learned as a child but can't follow through on the simplest of tasks, or something they were just asked to do.

Short-term memory—those events that just happened in the last few minutes—is the first type of memory that is damaged in dementia. If you're caring for someone with dementia, it is vitally important to think through all of the different ways loss of short-term memory will change someone's actions and behaviors. This loss of short-term memory often becomes a source of conflict for both the caregiver and the person with dementia.

- *"I asked Mom to do the dishes. She walked into the kitchen and then sat down and didn't do anything. Why won't she help out anymore?"*
- *"Dad said he was going to get me his checkbook, and the next thing I knew he was watching TV."*
- *"She keeps telling me I don't call. I've been calling her at least once a day."*
- *"My wife is accusing me of stealing her jewelry. Doesn't she realize that she keeps hiding it and then forgets where she put it?"*

In Chapter 9 we will look at strategies for working with memory loss that can help reduce conflict and emotional upsets. Bottom line, it's important to remember that the person with dementia is not intentionally forgetting things—no matter how frustrating this forgetfulness is for you.

Is short-term memory the same thing as recall?

"I asked Dad to do the dishes, and even had him repeat it back. But then I left the room for just a minute and he'd completely forgotten."

Through the early and even middle stages of dementia, people will be able to repeat things you've just said in the last few seconds: this is recall. However, if you wait a couple minutes and then ask them what you said, they will have forgotten: this is short-term memory.

This difference between recall and short-term memory demonstrates how the brain processes and remembers information. For a person with dementia, it's almost like their brain is a computer whose memory is no longer able to accept new information onto the hard drive for long-term storage.

Why does Mom remember some things some of the time?

Like the previous answer, this has to do with how our memory works, and how memory deteriorates in dementia. In the early and even middle stages of dementing illnesses, it's common for people to have days, minutes, and hours where they seem to be doing better. They remember things more clearly; after having forgotten your dog's name for the last month, they'll suddenly remember it. This brings up all kinds of questions for family members: "Are they getting better?," "Maybe they really don't have dementia?," and invariably, "Are they doing this on purpose?"

Memory, and our ability to recall things, varies even within people who don't have dementia. Different things can play into this day-to-day and minute-to-minute variability in our memory. Are we rested or tired? How stressed out and preoccupied are we? These factors have even more effect on someone with dementia.

There's also the phenomenon that people with dementia may remember topics of particular meaning and emotional importance more than other things—this is sometimes referred to as limbic memory, which refers to deep structures in the brain. If someone has always been concerned with money, they could surprise you—even with a moderate degree of dementia—and say, *"where's the twenty dollars you owe me?"* Or maybe religion has been a strong focus, and out of the blue the person with dementia will remind you, *"Aren't we supposed to light a candle for Father this week?"*

So while you will see subtle changes in the person's ability to remember—good days and bad days—it's important to remember that the person with Alzheimer's is not faking memory loss. If anything, they are frustrated and struggling to retrieve information and abilities that they are losing or have lost.

Why does my mother think her grandson is her son?

As a dementia progresses, it's common for people to confuse one close relative with another, especially someone from earlier in their life, such as a parent or sibling. This likely has to do with old memories staying longer than new ones, and facial similarities that have been passed along through the generations.

You may also be a spousal caregiver who is confused for a parent. One possible reason for this could be the caretaker role, in which you now help them with dressing, feeding, bathing, etc. These activities may remind the person with dementia of a much earlier time, when a parent performed these functions. In later stages of dementia, it's common that even close relatives and a spouse will no longer be recognized.

This mistaking and forgetting of identities can trigger a range of emotions and reactions in caregivers and family members—anger, sadness, loss, even humor and laughter. It's fine to gently correct the person, but you may or may not get the desired recognition. This mistaking of identities is part of the disease progressing.

What are instrumental activities of daily living (IADLs)?

- *"John has always kept the checkbook, but I just looked and it's all added wrong."*
- *"I was over at Mom's and she used to keep her desk and all the bills so neat; now it's just one big avalanche, and I found a whole stack of unpaid bills wedged behind the bookshelf."*

Instrumental activities of daily living (IADLs) refers to a broad range of skills people are able to do to maintain a household, finances, transportation, etc. Unlike the ADLs, which cover our most basic needs (see the following question), IADLs involve a greater level of thought and organization—though when we're well, we take doing these things for granted.

In progressive dementias it is usually the IADLs that are impaired first, followed by the ADLs. It is also common that relatives and spouses will notice problems with IADLs as one of the first signs of dementia.

Some IADLs are:
- Finances
  - Balancing a checkbook
  - Making change
  - Writing checks
  - Using an ATM
- Shopping
- Housework

- preparing a meal
- cleaning
- laundry
- Driving
- Overall functioning in a workplace
- Reading and writing
- Using public transportation
- Manage medications

What are activities of daily living (ADLs)?

Our ability to perform tasks is divided into two broad categories. The ADLs are our most basic skills. Loss of ADLs most often occurs after the higher-functioning IADLs have diminished, and it is often this loss of the ability to perform basic ADL tasks that results in caregivers no longer being able to keep their loved one in the home.

ADLs include:
- Bathing
- Eating
- Toileting
- Dressing
- Walking

What is mild cognitive impairment (MCI)?

Mild cognitive impairment (MCI) describes a condition that is in excess of the normal forgetfulness that can come with aging, yet is not to the level of a diagnosable dementia. The person with MCI is able to function in all spheres of their life, but they—and likely those close to them—have begun to notice problems with memory, attention, and possibly mood. Their thinking may have become rigid (unwilling to compromise or listen to other points of view) and they may be prone to repeating themselves.

- *"There's no reasoning with mother!"*
- *"Doesn't he know he's told that story ten times already?"*

People with MCI are at increased risk for developing full-blown Alzheimer's or another dementia; it may in fact be a very early form of dementia. However, others will remain stable, and for some—it is not known why—the symptoms will go away entirely.

What are the stages of dementia?

There are multiple staging systems for rating the severity of dementia, but there are four large, general stages that are universally agreed upon: mild cognitive impairment (which may not progress to dementia), early dementia, moderate dementia, and severe dementia. See the table beginning on page 16 for an explanation of each stage.

How long can someone live with Alzheimer's?

The average life expectancy from the time of diagnosis until death is seven to nine years, although people who are physically healthy may live twenty years or longer. While Alzheimer's disease was the fifth leading cause of death in 2004 for American adults over the age of sixty-five, many people with Alzheimer's and other dementias will ultimately die from other causes, such as pneumonia, heart attack, and stroke.

What are the risk factors for developing Alzheimer's?

The single-greatest risk for Alzheimer's disease, as well as vascular dementia, is age. By age sixty-five it's estimated that between 2–10 percent of people will have dementia, and this number doubles with approximately every five years of age. So by the time a person is in their mid-eighties, there is a 35–50 percent chance that they will have a moderate or greater degree of dementia.

Stages of Dementia

Stage	Changes in thinking (cognition)	Behavior and emotional changes	Changes in the ability to perform tasks	Score on Mini-Mental State Exam*
Mild cognitive impair-ment	Increased forgetfulness	Depression and anxiety are common. The person may become rigid in their thinking.	Still able to function in all areas— socially, occupa-tionally, and in the home.	26–30
Early dementia	Memory loss, especially for recent events, and problems learning new material. Speech may become repetitive and the same story told over and over. Increased diffi-culty with communicating, problems finding words. Difficulty making decisions.	Depression, anxiety, loss of interest in usual activities. Paranoia and hallucinations may occur. In some instances, there could be impulsive behavior or lack of initiative.	Mistakes and acci-dents common in balancing the check-book, driving a car, preparing meals.	20–26

...Continued

Stage	Changes in thinking (cognition)	Behavior and emotional changes	Changes in the ability to perform tasks	Score on Mini-Mental State Exam*
Moderate dementia	Memory worsens, including memory for more distant events and people. The ability to reason is lost. The person can only follow simple one-step instructions: "Chew your food." "Drink your juice."	Agitation and rapid changes in mood and behavior are common.	Only able to perform the most basic tasks.	10–20
Severe dementia	Total loss of memory, including being able to recognize relatives and spouse. The ability to comprehend and follow instructions is lost. Speech is mostly gone.	Extreme disturbance in both behavior and emotion. This can appear as either highly agitated behavior or totally flat, in which the person does absolutely nothing and can remain motionless for hours.	Requires complete assistance with all activities: bathing, toileting, eating, walking, and dressing.	0–10

*see Chapter 4 for description of the Mini-Mental State Exam (MMSE)

After age comes genetics—does Alzheimer's run in your family?

Increasingly, there is evidence that the same risk factors associated with developing heart disease and stroke may also increase the risk for developing dementia. This is especially true for blood pressure, and several studies have found that taking anti-hypertensive medication decreases the risk of developing Alzheimer's. Other treatable risk factors being studied include obesity, elevated cholesterol, and cigarette smoking.

On average, women live longer than men, so women may be at a slightly greater risk of developing Alzheimer's.

If I have a parent with Alzheimer's, what are the chances that I will develop it?

If you have a first-degree relative (mother, father, sister, brother) who had late-onset Alzheimer's, your risk goes up three to four times. If you had two or more first-degree relatives with Alzheimer's, your risk goes up more than sevenfold. The genetic risk is even higher for people who have relatives with early-onset Alzheimer's (Alzheimer's that develops before the age of sixty-five, most commonly in the fifties, but can occur as early as a person's thirties or forties).

Are there things you can do to prevent getting Alzheimer's?

There have been many studies and attempts to identify things that can protect us from developing Alzheimer's. However, as various studies' findings are reported, they're quickly picked up by the popular press and we're bombarded with information that may not be accurate or doesn't apply to our particular situation. Often, later studies come out and say the exact opposite—as happened with hormone-replacement therapy for women, which at one point was thought to decrease the incidence of dementia. In actuality, it was later discovered that women on hormone-replacement therapy may be at an increased risk for developing dementia.

The most encouraging data supports decreasing your risk of developing Alzheimer's by combating the avoidable contributing factors: treating hypertension and diabetes, watching your weight and your cholesterol level, not smoking, getting regular exercise, and eating a healthy diet. Additionally, multiple studies have reported that people with higher levels of education are at a decreased risk of developing dementia.

Another area of intense interest is the use of nonsteroidal anti-inflammatory drugs (NSAIDs), such as ibuprofen (Motrin, Advil) and Naprosyn. While it does not appear that these medications reverse or slow down the advance of Alzheimer's in people who already have symptoms, there is some evidence to support them decreasing the overall chances of developing Alzheimer's. Of course, regularly taking these medications carries other risks, such as stomach problems and ulcers.

Can dementia be cured?

In Chapter 5 we will review different forms of dementia, including those that are potentially reversible. However, the vast majority of dementia is not presently curable. Current medical treatments can help slow the advance of Alzheimer's and other dementias, but do not cure them. In Chapter 19 we will look at promising new experimental medical therapies that, though they may not be a cure, act more directly on the processes of cell damage and death in the brain that are believed to cause Alzheimer's.

If I am getting more forgetful, does that mean I'm going to develop Alzheimer's?

A certain amount of forgetfulness goes along with normal aging. The experience of forgetting where you left your keys or even your car in a crowded parking lot does not mean you are developing a dementia. This is sometime referred to as "benign forgetfulness of old age." It is different from early dementia and mild cognitive impairment (MCI), and is not a cause for worry. However, should there be emotional changes and/or impairment in a person's ability to perform everyday tasks, a medical evaluation should be sought.

Chapter 3

GETTING A DIAGNOSIS

- What symptoms signal a need for treatment?
- How do you get someone to go for an evaluation if they don't want to?
- What if one parent needs an evaluation, but the other refuses to have it done?
- How stressful is a dementia evaluation?
- My mother is easily upset; must we tell her she has Alzheimer's?
- How does someone get diagnosed with a dementia?
- What are the diagnostic criteria of dementia?
- How important is getting an accurate diagnosis?
- Who can diagnose dementia?
- What should I look for in a doctor or treatment team?
- Are there specialists who work with dementia?
- What role do family members play in getting an accurate diagnosis?
- What's delirium, and is it the same thing as dementia?
- What if I disagree with the diagnosis?
- Once a diagnosis is made, how often should someone be reevaluated?

What symptoms signal a need for treatment?

The answer to this depends on who is seeking treatment—the person with the dementia, or a concerned family member. If it's the patient, the symptoms that are likely to lead them to seek treatment may have nothing to do with memory loss, but more often center on emotional changes and physical complaints:

- *"I don't feel right."*
- *"I have no energy."*
- *"I'm depressed."*
- *"I'm constantly nervous."*
- *"Everything seems so much harder to do."*

If it's a family member or significant other who wants to bring the person to a clinician, chances are the symptoms are more extreme and will include problems with memory and behavioral and/or emotional changes.

- *"He hasn't paid his bills in four months."*
- *"He's had three fender benders with the car."*
- *"She sits alone in her apartment in the middle of the summer with no air-conditioning."*
- *"She keeps messing up her medications; I think maybe she's been taking too many."*

How do you get someone to go for an evaluation if they don't want to?

A point worth repeating is that it's important to step away from arguments with people who have dementia. They are not being deliberately obstinate or difficult. Try to keep in mind that they have brain damage, and part of what needs to be managed is how to get through the rough spots—one of which may be a trip to the doctor or the dementia clinic.

Even though the person with dementia may look absolutely normal, they are struggling with remembering things and how to complete more complex tasks. Changes in routine—such as a trip to the doctor—can seem overwhelming and bring out crippling anxiety. This negative response can be worsened by the caregiver's own fears and misgivings, many of which get communicated through facial expression, tone of voice, and non-verbal cues.

Things you can do to help get your loved one into the car and through the evaluation are:

- Be as calm as possible, even if you don't feel calm.
- Speak softly and in a low clear tone.
- Keep instructions and explanations simple. There's no need to say, "We're going to a specialty clinic for an evaluation of dementia." Instead it's probably best to say, "We're going to the doctor." Or, if you're caring for a person who has a greater degree of dementia and this invokes too much anxiety, "Let's go for a ride."
- When faced with an intense emotional response, try to gently distract the person from the thing that has them so upset. Once the outburst has passed, you can try again.
  - "Let's have some tea."
  - "Let's see what's on the TV."
  - Put on soothing music
  - Give them a snack or a drink.

What if one parent needs an evaluation, but the other refuses to have it done?

"Your father is just having a little trouble with forgetting things. Stop making such a big thing of it. It's no one's business but ours, and I wish you would butt out!"

This is a common situation that can have a number of twists. When one part of a married or committed couple develops dementia, it creates changes in all aspects of the relationship (discussed more thoroughly in Chapter 16). One response to these changes is the healthy spouse/partner trying to move forward as though nothing has happened. The reasons behind this can be complex and include feelings of depression, shame, denial, fear, and loss. The healthy spouse may feel quite strongly that they don't want to burden others, or that there is nothing to be gained from having their partner diagnosed.

- *"He's just a bit forgetful, that's all."*
- *"There's nothing wrong with her, please stay out of our business."*
- *"I don't want anyone to know."*

As the dementia worsens and it's less able to be hidden, the healthy spouse is at great risk for withdrawing from friends, family, their faith community, social clubs, etc.—the very supports that are so vital when caring for someone with dementia. Here are some good ways to approach the healthy spouse about seeking the necessary treatment for their partner with dementia:

- Be clear with your concerns, and state what you've actually witnessed—don't exaggerate. Avoid confrontation.
  - *"He couldn't add the check to figure the tip; he never had a problem with that before."*
  - *"He's forgetting to check the mirrors when he drives."*
  - *"He couldn't remember his granddaughter's name."*

Listen to the healthy spouse's concerns, and let them know that they've been heard.

Offer to make the appointment for the assessment, and tell them that you're willing to go along.

Provide education, such as this book or a smaller pamphlet like those available from the Alzheimer's Association.

Let them know you will be there for them, whatever the outcome. Instill hope.

- *"Many people go through this, there's more and more that can be done to help."*
- *"They have medications now that can slow it down."*

How stressful is a dementia evaluation?

A dementia evaluation itself is not all that stressful—the stress involved typically comes from the fear of being diagnosed with Alzheimer's. This stress is usually at its highest right before the appointment. However, the professionals who perform these evaluations—particularly if you go to a specialty clinic—have a wealth of information on the disease and are used to working with people with dementia and their caregivers. They have learned how to gently and kindly get people through the various tests and examinations.

The caregiver(s) and person with dementia will be provided with necessary information, and will have the opportunity to ask questions. You will be reassured that you are not alone and that millions of other families are going through something quite similar. (See the next chapter for specific information on what the evaluation entails.)

There is no doubt that the diagnosis of dementia and Alzheimer's carries a great deal of fear and a sense of loss. Over the course of your evaluation this bad news will be tempered with learning about practical ways to get through things and that there is hope.

My mother is easily upset; must we tell her she has Alzheimer's?

The answer to this question needs to be tailored to you and your situation. In earlier stages of dementia, it is likely that the person will be able to understand, remember, and process the diagnosis. The information will be important for them to have so that they can make the needed plans and participate as fully as possible in their treatment.

However, as short-term memory fails, it's unlikely that the information will be retained, and there is a real risk that the person will hear the news—even if it's not for the first time—and respond catastrophically. So, while honesty is usually the best policy, it may come down to a matter of kindness and practicality and you may decide not to burden your loved one with the diagnosis. Or, if they at one time knew their diagnosis, but have now forgotten it, there's little point in insisting they remember.

This strategy is sometimes called "therapeutic lying," and we will discuss it further in Chapter 7. Ultimately, it's an approach that places kindness first and it does take a bit of practice.

- *"Mom, the doctor says you're doing just fine."*
- *"Dear, you're just having a little problem with forgetfulness."*

How does someone get diagnosed with a dementia?

The diagnosis of dementia is based on family and patient history and physical, neurological, and psychiatric examinations and is supported through the use of blood work, brain imaging, and other tests as required. It is a clinical diagnosis that can be made with a high degree of accuracy—Alzheimer's disease can be diagnosed with roughly 90 percent certainty and vascular dementias are accurately diagnosed between 70–80 percent of the time.

While there are better diagnostic tests currently being studied for Alzheimer's, this disease cannot be 100 percent diagnosed in living people. The most accurate way to diagnose Alzheimer's is still after death, with an autopsy and brain examination.

What are the diagnostic criteria of dementia?

Commonly used diagnostic criteria for Alzheimer's disease and other dementias are those found in the Diagnostic and Statistical Manual (*DSM-IV-TR*), which is published by the American Psychiatric Association. The diagnosis of Alzheimer's is also often made using criteria established by the National Institute of Neurological and Communicative Disorders and Stroke-Alzheimer's Disease and Related Disorders Association (NINCDS-ADRDA).

In general, a diagnosis of dementia requires the loss of a prior level of functioning and ability in an otherwise alert and awake person. It will also include:

- Measurable loss of memory
- One or more other areas of loss in the brain's ability to function (cognition)
  - Language problems (aphasia):
    - Finding words
    - Understanding and following conversations
    - Speaking in a way that others can understand
    - Reading and comprehending
    - Writing and spelling
  - Problems carrying out physical tasks (apraxia):
    - Fastening buttons
    - Putting the right limb through the right opening in a garment
    - Putting garments on in the correct order
    - Holding utensils
    - Putting the cap on a tube of toothpaste
    - Getting into and out of a car
    - Putting on a seatbelt
  - Inability to recognize familiar objects and/or people (agnosia):
    - Forgetting what different things are called

- ❏ Forgetting names
- ❏ Forgetting relationships and how someone is connected to them
- ◆ Problems with tasks that involve planning and organizing (executive functions):
  - ❏ Keeping a checkbook
  - ❏ Planning a meal
  - ❏ Driving a car
  - ❏ Holding a job

There are also some physical diagnostic criteria; more on that in the next chapter.

How important is getting an accurate diagnosis?

Once you or your loved one has been diagnosed with a dementia, determining the type and/or cause becomes important. First, you will want to ensure that potentially reversible or stoppable causes of dementia have been ruled out, such as dementia caused by a head injury. Next, understanding the type of dementia will help steer you—and your treatment team—toward strategies that will be most effective and carry the lowest degree of risk.

Who can diagnose dementia?

The majority of dementia diagnoses will be made by primary care physicians, geriatricians, neurologists, and psychiatrists. In specialty clinics, the diagnosis might be made by an advanced practice nurse (APRN), psychologist, or neuropsychologist.

What should I look for in a doctor or treatment team?

Because most dementias are progressive and will continue over a number of years, you will want to have a doctor or team of professionals who will be with you and your loved one through the long haul. It's best to have someone who will be available—or have a back up—if you find yourself in the midst of a behavioral or medical crisis, whether big or small. You might be surprised by some of the things you'll want advice on:

- *"I think she's in pain, but she can't tell me where it is."*
- *"He's stopped eating."*
- *"She keeps trying to get out of the house."*
- *"She refuses to take a bath."*
- *"He keeps trying to take out the car."*

You will want someone who is experienced in treating dementia and with whom you are comfortable working closely. Ideally, your provider or treatment team will also have a good understanding of area resources and will be able to steer you to them according to what you need at the moment.

Are there specialists who work with dementia?

Around the country there are both dementia specialists and specialty clinics that focus solely on the treatment of dementia. Within the medical profession there are geriatric specialists (geriatricians), geriatric psychiatrists, and neurologists who focus on illnesses of later life. A specialty clinic will often include case managers, social workers, advanced practice nurses, and possibly physical and occupational therapists. These specialists can provide thorough evaluations and recommendations for strategies and treatments to address the behaviors and symptoms of your loved one. Specialty clinics are often, although not always, associated with medical schools and community hospitals.

What role do family members play in getting an accurate diagnosis?

Family members (including spouses and involved friends) are a vital part of any dementia evaluation. You are the ones who have observed the behaviors and symptoms. You'll be able to tell the professional when you first started to notice problems and whether or not the changes came on all at once, or if they happened in slow stages.

Many geriatric specialists will have family members complete questionnaires that ask about different symptoms. Some clinics will mail these out prior to the evaluation. These tools will frequently break down symptoms of dementia into three broad categories:

- Activities: What kinds of things is the person still able to do? What do they now require assistance with?
- Behavioral changes: Are there symptoms of depression, anxiety, or anger? Have there been tantrums, rage attacks, or loss of motivation? Does the person seem to repeat themselves, or engage in activities that have no apparent purpose (pacing, staring out a window, turning light switches on and off)?
- Thinking (cognition): What kinds of things are being forgotten? Do they struggle to find words? Do they have trouble speaking in clear sentences, or in understanding what others say to them?

Doctors will rely on you for a clear and accurate record of symptoms, which will help them make the correct diagnosis.

What's delirium, and is it the same thing as dementia?

A caregiver for someone with dementia needs to be on the lookout for sudden changes in a person's level of function, especially should they appear less awake and alert. Delirium is a medical term that describes a confused state, where the person's level of alertness is quite changeable and seems to wax and wane. They can be awake one minute and barely responsive the next. They may hallucinate, seeing things or hearing things that aren't real, and their behavior can become erratic. A delirium can come on fast or be slowly progressive. Delirium is not the same thing as dementia; up until the very late stages of dementing illnesses, people are awake and alert.

Many things—mostly medical—can cause delirium and people with dementia are at high risk for developing a delirium on top of their dementia. Should a delirium develop, getting prompt medical attention, finding its cause, and treating it are crucial. While thousands of things can cause a delirium, here are some of the more common causes:

- Problems with medications
  - Drug interactions
  - Too much or too little of a medication
- Medical problems
  - Blood sugar being either too high or too low
  - Problems with thyroid hormone
  - Constipation that has progressed to a total bowel obstruction
  - Stroke
  - Heart attack
- Infections
  - Urinary tract infections
  - Pneumonia
  - Bed sores
- Hospitalization
  - intensive care unit syndrome
  - after surgery (post-surgical) delirium

- Withdrawal syndromes
  - ◆ Withdrawal from alcohol (delirium tremens)
  - ◆ Withdrawal from sedative medications (benzodiazepines—Valium, Xanax, Ativan, etc.)
  - ◆ Withdrawal from other medications, including antidepressants

What if I disagree with the diagnosis?

It's common, especially in the earlier stages of a dementia, to desperately want the problems to be something other than progressive dementia. A thorough diagnostic evaluation should help rule out—or in—all of the various conditions that can cause the symptoms you or your loved one are experiencing. Still, in the early and even the moderate stages of dementia, symptoms can be severe one minute, and not so bad the next. It's normal for people to wonder if maybe the doctor wasn't right after all. Maybe it's a reaction to the medication, or they're just doing this to get attention, or…

But the bottom line is that coming to terms with the diagnosis is an important step so that you can move on with treatment and all of the planning that is best done sooner rather than later. However, as with any other condition, if you leave an evaluation feeling that the wrong diagnosis has been given, there are two basic things you can try: see if additional tests might better clarify the diagnosis, or get a second opinion. If both of these approaches indicate dementia, it's time to accept the diagnosis.

Once a diagnosis is made, how often should someone be reevaluated?

This will depend on the individual, their caregivers, and their symptoms. If things are going well, routine follow-up visits with the geriatric specialist or internist may be every three to six months. At that time, different strategies can be evaluated and follow-up testing obtained to see if the dementia has improved, stayed the same, or worsened.

If the person is not doing well and their symptoms are worsening, it's important to have them seen soon and possibly more frequently, in order to try and get things stabilized.

Chapter 4

THE DEMENTIA EVALUATION

- What information should I prepare for a family member's evaluation?
- How can I help the professionals with their evaluation?
- How important is getting an MRI or CT scan?
- What about other kinds of brain imaging, like PET and SPECT scans?
- When does someone need their brain waves mapped with an EEG?
- Will my father need to have a brain biopsy to get a diagnosis?
- Will a physical examination be necessary?
- Will vision and hearing need to be checked?
- What blood tests are part of the evaluation?
- Are there genetic tests for Alzheimer's?
- My mother developed Alzheimer's in her early fifties; should I get tested?
- Are there screening tests for dementia?
- What is the Mini-Mental State Examination?
- What kinds of psychological testing might be done in a dementia evaluation?

What information should I prepare for a family member's evaluation?

To maximize the usefulness of the evaluation, it's important to assemble as much information about your loved one as possible. At the minimum, this should include:

- A full medical history that includes:
  - Active medical conditions that are being treated
  - Past surgeries
  - Any known allergies or adverse reactions to medications
- Past psychiatric history
- A thorough list of all medications, including over-the-counter pills and nutritional supplements
- Social history
  - Who is in the family?
  - What kind of resources and insurance do they have?
- Social habits
  - Smoking
  - Alcohol intake
- Insurance Information (and remember to bring insurance cards)
- Prior level of functioning.
  - How far did the person go in school?
  - What kind of job did they/do they hold?
  - Hobbies?

How can I help the professionals with their evaluation?

Prior to a dementia evaluation, many clinics and geriatric specialists mail out lengthy questionnaires to family members. These often include checklists that go through an array of tasks and functions and ask whether or not the person is still able to complete them. Some break this down further and want to know if the person performs a given task by themselves, with a little help, or if they need total assistance. Common tests include the Blessed Dementia Scale and a user-friendly version of the Clinical Dementia Rating (CDR).

Many geriatric specialists and specialty clinics develop their own tools, such as the very thorough questionnaire in Appendix C, based on the one used at Yale-New Haven Hospital's Adler Geriatric Assessment Center. It's a good idea to go through this kind of written overview prior to any evaluation. It will help you think through the person's various strengths and problem areas, and will give the professionals a lot of useful information.

How important is getting an MRI or CT scan?

Most experts now recommend that some form of brain imaging be obtained in the course of a dementia evaluation. This will likely be either a computer tomography (CT) scan or magnetic resonance imaging (MRI). These images can help to identify likely causes of dementia and to rule out others. In general, an MRI offers a clearer picture, and can be particularly useful in identifying patterns of brain loss, old strokes, signs of an infection, bleeds, and other structural abnormalities.

One potential downside to MRIs is that many individuals find that these tests, which involve being placed inside a tube, invoke intense feelings of claustrophobia (fear of enclosed spaces). For someone who has an agitated dementia, staying still for half an hour while this test is performed may not be realistic.

What about other kinds of brain imaging, like PET and SPECT scans?

The world of brain imaging—and radiology in general—is going through a period of exciting and intense growth. It wasn't that long ago that we were confined to the static images of X-rays, CT scans, and regular MRIs. The past two decades have seen the development of "functional" imaging. Basically, this means that we're going from snapshots to motion pictures, and can actually observe how the brain uses various nutrients, such as sugar and oxygen, as well as other compounds. Positron emission tomography (PET), single-photon emission tomography (SPECT), and functional MRIs are all being used as research tools to better understand the changes that occur in the brain during all the different dementias.

At present these tests are not part of a routine dementia evaluation. However, if there is uncertainty as to a diagnosis, these tests may be used. It is likely that as these become more available and affordable, they will become a part of the standard workup.

When does someone need their brain waves mapped with an EEG?

People with dementia will often have abnormal brain-wave findings on an electroencephalograph (EEG). Usually this takes the form of an overall slowing in brain wave activity. In general, an EEG is not part of the standard dementia evaluation, but may be requested to help clarify a diagnosis, or if the person has a history of seizures.

Will my father need to have a brain biopsy to get a diagnosis?

No. While it is true that an absolute diagnosis of Alzheimer's disease can currently only be obtained through a biopsy (piece of tissue) taken from the brain, this usually occurs after the person has passed away, at autopsy. Because of the significant risk involved in doing this while a person is alive (bleeding, infection, stroke), and the relative accuracy of noninvasive, clinical diagnosis, a brain biopsy is not performed as part of a typical dementia evaluation.

Will a physical examination be necessary?

A physical examination is a standard part of any dementia evaluation. In the course of the physical, the doctor, nurse practitioner (APRN), or physician's assistant (PA) will pay particular attention both to the broad range of physical symptoms that can help diagnose a particular form of dementia and to symptoms that may worsen an existing dementia.

Areas of particular interest will include:

- Elevated blood pressure—associated with strokes and vascular dementia
- Abnormal heart rhythms—this can put the person at an increased risk for having blood clots
- A thorough neurologic examination looking for physical signs of past stroke—these might include a limp, facial droops, abnormal reflexes, specific problems in understanding or using language, muscle weakness, etc.

Will vision and hearing need to be checked?

While vision and hearing examinations may not be part of the dementia evaluation, it's a good idea to get both of these done. As we age, problems with hearing loss and visual changes are common. Additionally, eye disorders, such as cataracts, glaucoma, and macular degeneration can further impair the functioning of a person with dementia.

Making sure your loved one has the right glasses and/or hearing aids will improve their overall well-being and ability to function. As the dementia progresses, simple strategies to keep these aids handy—such as keeping eyeglasses on a necklace, having multiple pairs, and regularly checking the battery on hearing aids—will be important to the patient's comfort.

What blood tests are part of the evaluation?

A typical dementia evaluation will include having a few tubes of blood drawn. Specific tests include:

- A complete blood count (CBC). This will show whether or not the person is anemic, and may reveal subtle signs of nutritional deficiencies (vitamin B12 and folate) that can cause or worsen dementia. Certain abnormalities in the CBC may give evidence that a person has been a long-time drinker, or that they have an infection.
- Electrolytes—these are the salts (sodium, potassium, chloride, and bicarbonate) dissolved in our bloodstream. Electrolyte abnormalities can be the sign of many diseases and can also be related to medication side effects, as is sometimes seen with people on certain blood-pressure pills (diuretics) whose potassium can drop to dangerous levels.
- Liver function tests
- Tests to evaluate the health of the kidneys
- Thyroid-function tests—to rule out abnormalities, such as having too little thyroid hormone (hypothyroidism), which can look like a dementia.
- Tests to check the levels of folic acid (folate) and vitamin B12
- Sedimentation rate—a test that measures the speed with which red blood cells sink in a tube of blood. A rate that's too high can be an indicator of a chronic inflammatory illness, such as arthritis.

Other tests that are commonly obtained may include:
- A test to rule out syphilis
- HIV test

Are there genetic tests for Alzheimer's?

Genetic testing (the examination of a person's DNA) for dementia is an area of active research, and three genes have been identified in the development of Alzheimer's. However, genetic testing is not typically part of a routine dementia assessment. It's most likely recommended for those forms of dementia that are clearly passed on (autosomal dominant or recessive). This will include early-onset Alzheimer's and Huntington's disease, but not later-onset Alzheimer's or vascular dementias, where the genetic, inherited component is less clear.

My mother developed Alzheimer's in her early fifties; should I get tested?

There are strong and emotionally powerful reasons that bring someone in for genetic testing. If you believe that you are at significant risk for developing a dementia—such as early-onset Alzheimer's or Huntington's—a negative result can drastically reduce anxiety and may guide important life decisions, such as whether or not to have children.

A test that reveals an increased likelihood that you will develop a serious disorder can be both emotionally devastating and empowering. Someone who realizes that they have limited years of good health may find that this knowledge kicks them into gear. On a more practical level, many people at risk for inherited dementias want the answer so that they can make appropriate planning for their loved ones—getting wills in order, setting up a trust (see chapter 13), appointing a medical decision maker, power of attorney, etc.

Are there screening tests for dementia?

There are a number of screening tests that can help determine if someone has dementia. These examination tools, which are like verbal and written quizzes, typically take between five to fifteen minutes to complete. They quickly look at various areas of brain functioning, especially ones that are most often involved in dementing illnesses—memory, different aspects of understanding and using language, concentration, eye-hand coordination, and general orientation. The tests involve such questions as "What is your name?" "Where are you?" and "What's the date?"

The most-often-used screening test is the Folstein Mini-Mental State Examination (see the following question). Other question-naires, such as the Montreal Cognitive Assessment Tool (MoCA) are especially useful in either ruling out or diagnosing mild cogni-tive impairment. A positive screening test should always be followed up with a more thorough evaluation, as outlined in this chapter.

What is the Mini-Mental State Examination?
The Folstein Mini-Mental State Examination (MMSE) is the most commonly used screening tool for the evaluation of dementia. It has also been used extensively as a research tool when evaluating the benefits of different therapies and medications.

The evaluation takes between five to ten minutes to perform and each of the questions addresses a particular cognitive function of our brain. Items on the MMSE include:
- Orientation: Does the person know the day, date, year, month, season, where they are, the floor they are on, the city, county, and state? (10 points)
- Recall and Short-term memory: Can the person recall three items (3 points) and then remember them three to five minutes later? (3 points)
- Concentration: This usually involves having the person subtract backwards from 100 by 7 for a total of five times—

100, 93, 86, 79, 72. If the person can't do math, they will be asked to spell the word "world" backwards. (5 points)

- Can the person follow a command with multiple parts? "I want you to pick up a piece of paper in your right hand, fold it in half and then place it on the floor with your left hand." (3 points)
- Language:
  - ◆ The person is shown a sentence and asked to do what it says. Typically, the sentence is "Close your eyes." (1 point)
  - ◆ Write a sentence of your choice. (1 point)
  - ◆ Identify two common items. (2 points)
  - ◆ Repeat a simple sentence. (1 point)
- Eye-hand coordination (visuospatial). The person is shown a drawing of two intersecting five-sided figures and asked to copy it. (1 point)

The maximum score is 30.
- A score of 28–30 is considered normal.
- 26–28 may reveal signs of pre-dementia or mild cognitive impairment.
- 20–26 is mild dementia.
- 10–20 moderate dementia.
- Less than 10 is severe dementia.

What kinds of psychological testing might be done in a dementia evaluation?

While not always a part of a standard dementia evaluation, further psychological testing—neuropsychological testing—can be quite helpful in better assessing what kinds of things the person is still able to do. It may also be useful in clarifying a diagnosis. Neuropsychological testing is performed by a psychologist and will likely take a number of hours, possibly broken up into multiple sessions. The tests may include memory tasks, looking at ways in which the person solves problems, their verbal abilities, eye-hand coordination, and so forth.

To get the most out of this additional evaluation it will be important to review the findings with the psychologist and to think of practical ways the information can help. In particular you'll want to understand what things you, or your loved one, still do well and how these can be used to work around areas of decreased ability.

Chapter 5

ALZHEIMER'S AND OTHER TYPES OF DEMENTIA

- What are the major causes of dementia?
- What is Alzheimer's disease?
- How many people have Alzheimer's disease?
- What is the difference between early-onset and late-onset Alzheimer's?
- Who was Alzheimer?
- What causes Alzheimer's disease?
- Who gets Alzheimer's disease?
- What are vascular dementia and multi-infarct dementia?
- Does a vascular dementia manifest differently than Alzheimer's?
- Are there risk factors for vascular dementias?
- What is dementia with Lewy bodies?
- What is Parkinson's dementia?
- What is HIV dementia?
- What is frontal temporal dementia (Pick's disease)?
- Are some forms of dementia curable or reversible?
- What is alcohol dementia?
- Can alcohol dementia be treated?
- If my husband stops drinking will the alcohol dementia go away?
- What is pseudodementia of depression?
- What is neurosyphilis?
- What is normal pressure hydrocephalus?
- What else can cause dementia?

What are the major causes of dementia?

While there are over a hundred potential causes of dementia, these are the most frequent:

- Alzheimer's disease
- Vascular dementias (including multi-infarct/post-stroke dementia)
- Dementia with Lewy bodies
- Parkinson's associated dementia
- Frontal temporal dementia (Pick's disease)
- AIDS-related dementia
- Alcohol-related dementia (Korsakoff's syndrome)

What is Alzheimer's disease?

Alzheimer's is a progressive dementing illness that involves the destruction of brain cells. While the exact cause of the damage is not completely understood, there are two telltale lesions found in the brains of people with Alzheimer's.

- Neurofibrillary plaques—abnormal deposits of amyloid protein between nerve cells.
- Tangles—abnormal deposits of the tau protein inside brain cells (neurons).

In its earliest stages, symptoms include a decrease in short-term memory and forgetfulness, often accompanied by a diminished ability to find words. Emotional and personality changes in the early stages can include depression, anger, and paranoia. As the disease progresses, the memory loss becomes severe and may be accompanied by marked disturbances in behavior and emotion; the ability to reason is lost. In its final stages a person is unable to perform most tasks and requires total assistance with feeding, bathing, and basic hygiene.

How many people have Alzheimer's disease?

Alzheimer's disease is by far the most common cause of dementia in the United States—roughly two-thirds of all cases. It is estimated that anywhere from four-and-a-half to more than five million Americans are living with Alzheimer's, and it was the seventh leading cause of death in 2004.

What is the difference between early-onset and late-onset Alzheimer's?

Early-onset Alzheimer's affects people in their forties to sixties, and in rare instances can even develop in someone's thirties. This contrasts with the more common form of the disease, which doesn't occur until someone is in their late-sixties, seventies, eighties, or beyond. Another major difference is that early-onset dementia has a stronger genetic link—it is more likely to run in families or be autosomal dominant. This means that it only takes one of your parents to pass along the gene for you to get it. Early-onset accounts for a relatively small number of cases (about 5 percent) and is associated with mutations on three specific genes on chromosomes 1, 14, and 21. An interesting finding is that people with Down's syndrome, which in most cases is caused by having an extra chromosome 21, will almost all have Alzheimer's by the age of forty.

Who was Alzheimer?

Alois Alzheimer (1864–1915) was a German physician and researcher with a special interest in mental disorders, particularly dementia. In 1907 he published a short paper that described the microscopic findings (histology) in the brain of his patient Auguste D., a woman in her fifties with a severe and progressive dementia who had been brought to him for treatment six years earlier. In his carefully prepared and stained slides of brain tissue, Alzheimer revealed for the first time the neurofibrillary plaques and tangles that are the hallmarks of this disease. He also demonstrated that this form of dementia was different—at least on the microscopic level—from dementia caused by vascular disease.

What causes Alzheimer's disease?

Over the years there have been competing theories as to what causes Alzheimer's. Increasingly, the focus of interest is on deposits of amyloid in the brain; amyloid is a protein found in the plaques in the brain associated with Alzheimer's. Many researchers believe that it is the abnormal deposits of this protein that are responsible for the cell death seen in Alzheimer's. There is significant evidence to support this hypothesis, including the development of a genetically engi-neered mouse model with amyloid plaques that showed signs of dementia. In a very exciting study in 1999, these plaques were able to be reversed through the use of immunotherapy (see chapter 19), resulting in improvement in the functioning of these mice. The entire process by which amyloid is made and broken down by the body (amyloid cascade) is currently under intense investigation, and researchers are actively searching for ways to short-circuit the abnormal accumulation of this protein.

Apolipoprotein E (APOE), a protein involved in bringing lipids (fats) into the cell, has also been implicated in Alzheimer's. Different forms of this protein, which is coded on chromosome 19, have been shown to increase or decrease the risk of developing the disease. One form of this protein, called APOE-e4, has been shown to increase the risk by as much as fifteen times in Caucasians.

Who gets Alzheimer's disease?

With the exception of early-onset Alzheimer's (which accounts for 5 percent of cases), this is a disease of advancing age—all elderly people are susceptible to it. While some studies have questioned if women are at a slightly greater risk, this has not been proven. It affects all races, but studies suggest that Caucasians are more likely to contract Alzheimer's, while people of Asian descent are more likely to develop the vascular or multi-infarct form of dementia.

What are vascular dementia and multi-infarct dementia?

Vascular dementias are a group of conditions caused by either large or small strokes. These strokes can result from bleeding (hemorrhages), blood clots (embolus), blockage of blood vessels through the formation of plaques (thrombosis), or lack of oxygen to regions of the brain from other causes. The net result of all these causes is that key regions of the brain go without oxygen, and cell death—ischemia—results. Following the stroke(s), symptoms of dementia develop.

After Alzheimer's disease, vascular dementias account for the largest number of cases of dementia—roughly 20 percent, or one million Americans. There are also a large number of people—perhaps another million—who will have a combination of Alzheimer's and vascular dementia; this is called a "mixed dementia."

The most common form of vascular dementia is multi-infarct dementia.

Does a vascular dementia manifest differently than Alzheimer's?

There are several differences between vascular dementias and Alzheimer's disease that will be used when trying to make an accurate diagnosis.

- Vascular dementias often have a sudden onset, and progress in abrupt stages. This differs from Alzheimer's, which has a slow onset and steady progression.

- Loss of higher functioning (reasoning, shopping, handling finances, driving, doing housework, retrieving information, etc.) and the ability to perform basic self-care tasks can be lost rapidly in vascular dementia. This occurs more slowly in Alzheimer's.
- On brain imaging—CT scan or MRI—there will be evidence of strokes or small-blood-vessel disease in patients with vascular dementia. Brain images of people with Alzheimer's tend to show more diffuse patterns of brain-matter loss.
- Patients with vascular dementia may have a history of prior stroke(s).
- There is a greater likelihood of high blood pressure in patients with vascular dementias.
- General unsteadiness and frequent falls are more common with vascular dementia.
- Marked emotional and behavioral changes—depression, loss of motivation, sudden bursts of anger, inappropriate sexual behavior and/or language—may reflect damage to particular parts of the brain in a person with a vascular dementia.
- Patients with vascular dementia will often show specific neurological loss from their strokes. This could be:
  - Weakness or numbness in a limb, side of the body, or face
  - Specific deficits in understanding and expressing language (receptive and expressive aphasias)
  - A change in gait—this may take the form of small steps or a swinging-leg limp from weakness on one side of the body.
  - Loss of the ability to swallow

However, where as many as 20 percent of people with dementia will have both conditions, these differences may not always be clear. Further testing, including brain imaging, may be required to clarify diagnosis.

Are there risk factors for vascular dementias?

Risk factors for developing a vascular dementia are the same things that increase a person's likelihood of having a stroke. They include:

- High blood pressure (hypertension)
- Abnormal heart rhythms (cardiac arrhythmias), especially atrial fibrillation, which can predispose a person to blood clots if it's left untreated
- Sleep apnea (a condition where people will stop breathing for periods of time while they are asleep)
- Cigarette smoking
- Diabetes
- Coronary artery disease
- Abnormally elevated lipids, such as cholesterol (hyperlipidemia)

What is dementia with Lewy bodies?

Lewy bodies are abnormal brain cells, named after the man who discovered them. They can be associated with Alzheimer's disease, the dementia found in Parkinson's disease, and a disorder called dementia with Lewy bodies. Some researchers believe that Lewy body dementia—and not vascular dementia—is the second-leading cause of dementia in this country.

The symptoms of Lewy body dementia can be quite different from those of Alzheimer's, though sometimes the two conditions may be difficult to distinguish. Lewy body dementia occurs in later life (ages sixty to ninety) and it is progressive. Symptoms may include:

- Fluctuating levels in the ability to think straight. Attention and focus can be fine one moment and then the person drifts off, or loses track of what they were doing.
- Loss of coordination.
- Visual hallucinations. These can be very specific and quite real to the person having them.

- ◆ *"There's a little girl in a blue dress sitting on top of the television."*
- ◆ *"There are four red monkeys playing in the front lawn."*
- Sleep disturbances, such as rapid-eye-movement (REM) sleep disorder
  - ◆ The person may experience vivid dreams and act them out physically in their sleep. They will likely be unaware of this.
- Symptoms of Parkinson's disease
  - ◆ A slow, shuffling gait
  - ◆ Diminished facial expression, sometimes referred to as "mask-like"
  - ◆ Stiffness throughout the body, especially in the arms and legs

Unlike Alzheimer's, the memory loss with Lewy body dementia typically occurs later in the disorder. People with Lewy body dementia are also extremely sensitive to the side effects of anti-psychotic medications (discussed in Chapter 8). These medications are best avoided, or if they must be used to control disabling psychosis, they should be taken in the lowest possible dose.

What is Parkinson's dementia?

Parkinson's disease, a brain disorder that involves the destruction of nerve cells rich in the chemical messenger dopamine, carries a high rate of associated dementia. Eighty percent of people with Parkinson's will have some degree of dementia within eight years of diagnosis. The symptoms of Parkinson's dementia are very similar to Lewy body dementia, with prominent disturbances—including sometimes violent movements—during dream (REM) sleep, problems with attention, alertness, and concentration, and later onset of memory loss. The person will also demonstrate the physical symptoms of Parkinson's disease, including stiffness, decreased facial expression, and a slow shuffling gait. Some researchers consider

Lewy body dementia and Parkinson's dementia to be closely related conditions. Treatment recommendations are similar for both.

What is HIV dementia?

The HIV virus travels to the brain soon after infection, where it is taken up into the nerve cells. There it can cause a variety of damage, even in individuals who do not have full-blown AIDS. Since the onset of the HIV/AIDS epidemic, we have seen a range of dementia syndromes in people infected with the virus.

Early symptoms may be mild, and can include memory loss, problems with physical coordination (unsteadiness, dropping things,) tiredness, depression, psychosis, and even mania. As the dementia progresses, the memory loss and problems with coordination become severe and disabling. The individual becomes very slow in their movements and is unable to perform basic tasks.

What is frontal temporal dementia (Pick's disease)?

In the late 1900s, Dr. Arnold Pick described a form of dementia with profound disruption of speech (aphasia) and loss of inhibition, where people would begin to behave in ways that were impulsive and not characteristic of them. A specific lesion in the brain causing this form of dementia was later identified by Alois Alzheimer, and these legions became known as Pick bodies.

Areas of the brain most affected in this disorder are the frontal and temporal (sides) of the brain, and as such Pick's disease was eventually renamed frontal temporal dementia to more accurately reflect the disorder. It affects younger individuals and accounts for half of the cases of dementia in people under the age of sixty.

There are different types of frontal temporal dementia, and the symptoms can range from subtle to dramatic, and can include radical changes in a person's behavior and emotions. Someone who was previously quite restrained may suddenly start telling lewd jokes, or become sexually promiscuous. Or someone who used to be quite outgoing and had a great zest for life may suddenly seem depressed and apathetic.

Another common presentation of frontal temporal dementia involves prominent impairment of speech and language. The person will have trouble finding words and be unable to understand what others are saying. They may start talking in a strange fashion, and other language-related functions, such as reading and writing, will progressively deteriorate.

Are some forms of dementia curable or reversible?

The quick answer is "yes," but unfortunately the actual number of cases of dementia that reverse is quite small—less than 1 percent. However, there are a number of causes of dementia that, if treated, will not worsen; this happens in 10–15 percent of cases. This is one of the reasons why getting an early and accurate diagnosis is so important. The following questions in this chapter will review some causes of dementia that fall into this category.

What is alcohol dementia?

This is a form of dementia that affects long-time heavy drinkers, people who have done at least twenty years of heavy drinking. People with alcohol dementia, also known as Korsakoff's syndrome, will often try to cover for their lapses in memory by making things up (confabulation). As with other forms of dementia, because social functioning is preserved, the person with dementia may not be accurately diagnosed until the illness has progressed from mild to moderate. One feature of alcohol dementia that is a bit different from Alzheimer's disease is the early loss of the ability to learn and retain new information. While this also occurs in Alzheimer's, it is especially severe in the person with an alcohol dementia.

Can alcohol dementia be treated?
The best treatment is to get the person to stop drinking. If they were a daily drinker, they should seek medical supervision when they quit: They may be at risk for a serious and potentially life-threatening withdrawal syndrome, should they just stop cold turkey. In its most severe form, this withdrawal is known as delirium tremens— the "DTs"—and can include confusion, hallucinations, dangerous elevations in blood pressure, seizures, coma, and even death. Detoxification from alcohol can be safely managed with medications and typically takes between a few days and a couple of weeks. This detoxification is most safely handled on an inpatient unit, especially if the person with alcohol dementia has any history of seizures or withdrawal symptoms when they stop drinking.

If my husband stops drinking will the alcohol dementia go away?
If you can get the person to stop drinking, the alcohol dementia, unless it is accompanied by a second form of dementia such as Alzheimer's or vascular, should not get worse. Over the course of the first year away from alcohol it is common to see some improvement in the person's overall level of functioning, but it is unlikely they will return to their prior level of functioning.

What is pseudodementia of depression?
This term is somewhat controversial. Clinical depression can include symptoms of mental slowing, decreased speech, a loss of interest in usual activities, and poor concentration that may make the individual appear to have a dementia. When the depression is

treated, or goes away on its own, this "pseudo" or false dementia resolves.

However, some researchers looking into this phenomenon of pseudodementia, especially in older individuals, have shown that it is probably an early symptom of dementia, and that the majority of these people who are initially diagnosed with pseudodementia of depression go on to develop Alzheimer's disease and other dementias. This finding goes along with the related observation that many people with early dementia who seek treatment on their own come in with complaints of depression and anxiety. Also, when tested, most of these people will have some amount of memory loss, which is unrelated to their depressed mood.

What is neurosyphilis?

Prior to the 1940s, the sexually transmitted disease syphilis was the most common cause of dementia in the United States. In the nineteenth and early twentieth century, this form of dementia also accounted for the greatest number of people in psychiatric hospitals. Neurosyphilis went by a number of names, including general paralysis of the insane and dementia paralytica. This form of dementia occurred in the later stages of syphilis, after the person had been infected for a number of years. The majority of cases were with people in their mid-thirties through their fifties—quite a bit younger than the typical person with Alzheimer's. Similar to other progressive dementias, the symptoms start slowly and progress to profound and disabling problems with memory, other thought processes, behavior, and the ability to perform basic tasks and self-care activities. An unsteady gait can also be a symptom of neurosyphilis (ataxia/tabes dorsalis).

Since the development of antibiotics—penicillin in particular—that can cure syphilis, it has been rare to find cases of syphilis dementia. Even so, it is common to test for the organism that causes syphilis (treponema pallidum) when getting a dementia evaluation. If treated, the symptoms of neurosyphilis should not worsen, and some improvement may occur in the months and years following treatment. The near-elimination of neurosyphilis carries important messages. In this case, the discovery of a cure—penicillin—combined with early intervention before the brain is damaged, can prevent a person from developing a dementing illness.

What is normal pressure hydrocephalus?

Hydrocephalus, which literally means water on the brain, is a condition where spinal fluid (the fluid that cushions and nourishes the brain) becomes excessive. In normal pressure hydrocephalus (NPH), the brain fluid does not flow through the central nervous system (brain and spinal cord) as it normally would. As the fluid builds up it compresses and destroys brain tissue—when seen on a CT scan or MRI, the hollow chambers (ventricles) of an afflicted brain appear larger than normal.

NPH accounts for a small percent of dementia (less than 5 percent), and can be caused by head trauma, bleeding inside the head, infections, or the cause may not be known. The symptoms of NPH include dementia, an abnormal gait, changes in speech, and loss of bladder control. If caught early, NPH can be treated or its progression halted, through the use of a shunt that bypasses whatever is obstructing the flow of spinal fluid.

What else can cause dementia?

The list of rarer causes of dementia is lengthy, but it can be broken down into large categories. The following list does not include all of the possible causes of dementia, but it illustrates one of the reasons why getting an accurate diagnosis and not assuming that a dementia is Alzheimer's is important.

- Infections
  - HIV/AIDs
  - Syphilis
  - Whipple's disease
  - Lyme disease
  - Creutzfeld-Jakob disease (mad cow disease)
- Tumors
- Hormone disorders (endocrine)
- Head trauma
- Other neurological disorders
  - Huntington's disease
  - Multiple sclerosis
- Medication or drug-induced dementias
- Vitamin deficiencies
  - Vitamin B12 deficiency
  - Folic acid deficiency (vitamin B9)
  - Pellagra—niacin deficiency (vitamin B3)
- Other disorders
  - Down's syndrome

Chapter 6

TREATMENTS

What roles do family or other caregivers play in treatment?

The roles of the caregiver, whether you're a family member, close friend, or hired professional such as a private duty nurse, are central, varied, and change over time. As the person with dementia loses the ability to provide for herself, it will be up to you to do the thinking and planning. You will be placed in a variety of roles—advocate, friend, care-coordinator, legal guardian, financial planner, medical decision maker—and these will change with time and circumstance.

Not every treatment is for every person, and assessing what works and what doesn't is one of the most important, and at times difficult, caregiver roles. You, along with the person with dementia, are at the center of the treatment team. Your voices need to be heard and your concerns listened to. If something is not working, or you think it is making things worse, you need to make this clear. If it's a medication or other medical therapy, the prescribing physician or advanced practice nurse needs to be informed so that the treatment can be reviewed and modified as needed.

What is a care plan or treatment plan?

Treatment plans—sometimes called care plans—are based on the individual's current problems, strengths, and needs. Treatment plans serve a number of important purposes and as a caregiver or a person with dementia—even though you may not be a medical professional—it's good to know what's on them and to be involved in what goes into them. Different professionals involved in care will have their own treatment plans.

The plan includes the various services that are being recommended, what they are supposed to accomplish, how often they will be provided, and in what time frame these goals and objectives should be accomplished. Examples of services on a treatment plan might include:

- A visiting nurse to provide an in-home safety assessment that will take one to two hours, with ongoing updates as needed
- Medications X and Y as directed, to slow progression of disease
- Physical therapy twice weekly for one hour to increase mobility and help the patient learn to use her walker in a safe and consistent manner

Most insurers, including Medicare and Medicaid, insist that treatment plans are written and updated within a specified time frame, typically every three to six months. In order for providers—doctors, therapists, visiting nurses, in-home aides—to get paid for services delivered, there must be a treatment plan.

How do I know what kinds of treatment will be best for my wife?

Treatment of Alzheimer's and most other dementias needs to center on the person who has dementia and her family and caregiver(s). For the purpose of this book, the word "treatment" refers to any strategy or intervention that will help improve or stabilize how your loved one—and you—are doing. This "person-centered" approach provides the direction you'll need in figuring out the kinds of strategies that make sense for you. A person-centered approach includes some basic questions. How you answer them will help you identify treatments that are more likely to be effective.

Because of the progressive nature of most dementias, your answers will change over time. Also, don't be put off by the size of the list; it's often helpful to start with the area of immediate concern and then move on from there.

- What strengths does this person have? How can we take advantage of these?
  - *"My dad has a beautiful happy disposition even though he has advanced dementia."*

- ◆ *"My wife's physical health is pretty good."*
- ◆ *"You can give Mom a bowl of potatoes or apples and she'll peel for hours."*
- ◆ *"My brother just wants to be outside. He'll putter in the garden and be happy as a clam."*
- What strengths do you as a caregiver(s) have and how will these help?
  - ◆ *"I have a flexible work schedule."*
  - ◆ *"There are a lot of us to split up the duties of looking after Mom."*
  - ◆ *"I can afford some out-of-pocket care."*
  - ◆ *"I'm not easily flustered."*
  - ◆ *"I'm very organized."*
- What are the advantages and disadvantages of the current living situation?
  - ◆ *"She's unsteady in the bathroom."*
  - ◆ *"He keeps wanting to cook."*
  - ◆ *"He runs away every chance he gets."*
  - ◆ *"We've got a fenced-in backyard where he loves to garden."*
- What areas of mental functioning are impaired or lost?
  - ◆ Memory, concentration, the ability to perform complex or simple tasks, the ability to manage basic self-care such as bathing, dressing, feeding, etc.
- What areas of physical functioning are impaired or lost and what will help stabilize or improve these?
  - ◆ How steady are they on their feet; do they get lightheaded; do they have problems running out of breath and getting winded? Have there been falls?
- What are the active medical issues and what do we need to do to get them addressed?
- What gives this person, and you, the caregiver, pleasure, meaning, and joy and how can we maximize these types of activities?

- What behaviors are causing problems and what strategies will help reduce them?
  - *"She's always crying."*
  - *"He won't eat."*
  - *"He has terrible tantrums."*
  - *"She keeps wandering away from home."*
  - *"She won't stop smoking and there are burn marks all over the rug and furniture."*

What types of treatments are there?

Using the broad definition of treatment—anything that will help stabilize or improve the overall situation for you and your loved one—we can break down the options into two large categories, non-medical and medical, although there is some overlap.

Medical treatments and interventions might include:

- Medications (see Chapter 8)
- Treatment of active medical problems
- Regular vision and hearing assessments
- In-home nursing care
- Use of durable medical equipment such as walking and mobility aids (canes, walkers, wheelchairs), and other assistive equipment to help in the home (bath chairs, commodes, railings, a riser chair, etc.)

Non-medical interventions and treatments might include:

- Behavioral approaches to problem behaviors (see Chapter 9)
- Occupational and/or physical therapy
- Adult day care
- An emergency call system, including a button the person can press if they have a fall or are in need of emergency assistance
- A plan to manage wandering
- Music therapy

- Massage therapy
- Activity therapy
  - ◆ Art
  - ◆ Recreational activities
- Movement and dance
- Exercise
- Regularly scheduled activities
- Non-medication strategies to improve sleep
- Respite stays in a convalescent home (see Chapter 16)
- Home health aides
- Social work services
- Support groups

Will any treatments reverse Alzheimer's?

At present the answer is mostly no, although some individuals may experience a mild improvement of symptoms with the cholinesterase inhibitors donepezil, galantamine, rivastigmine (medications are discussed in Chapter 8). Current medication therapies act more to slow the progression of the illness—at least for a while—than to significantly reverse it. That said, there are exciting new treatments currently being tested that may reverse at least some portion of the disease.

However, the treatments that are discussed in this chapter mostly deal with improving the quality of life for both the person affected and the caregiver, and ensuring that the person with dementia is as safe and healthy as possible. These can be just as important—if not more so—than medication.

Are there differences in the treatment of Alzheimer's and vascular dementia?

At present, there are few differences in the medical treatment of Alzheimer's dementia and the vascular dementias. In both conditions you want to make sure that any risk factors for worsening of the disease—high blood pressure, elevated cholesterol, diabetes, etc.—are adequately controlled. This is especially important for vascular dementia.

As there is considerable overlap between these conditions—people with Alzheimer's often have some degree of vascular dementia and vice versa—it's common for people with diagnoses of a vascular dementia to be put on the same medications that have the FDA indication for the treatment of Alzheimer's, such as the cholinesterase inhibitors and memantine (Namenda).

How important is overall medical care?

While dementia is caused by diseases of the brain, the rest of the body can be relatively healthy. In general, people do better overall when they are physically well, and this is no different for a person with dementia. It's important to schedule regular checkups for existing medical problems, such as high blood pressure, arthritis, diabetes, etc., to make sure they are in control. In addition, you'll need to keep an eye out for emerging problems that, when small, may be easily treated, but if left too long can progress to something serious and disabling.

What other medical problems should we address?

The quick answer is that all medical problems need to be addressed. Included in the equation for good medical care are the following:

- Regular physical examinations that include routine lab work (complete blood count, electrolytes, and tests that look at the health of various organs such as the liver and kidneys)
- Regular vision and hearing tests—problems with sight and vision can worsen confusion and decrease function.
- Make sure that all prescribing physicians or advanced practice nurses are aware of every medication, including vitamins and

other nutritional supplements, the person is taking. A common problem is that when you have multiple prescribers, medications can get added without fully assessing any possible interactions.

- Pay attention to any problems walking, and be alert for the development of any sores on the person's feet—especially if they have poor circulation or diabetes. Great care needs to be exercised when trimming the toenails, and a visit to a podiatrist if problems develop—such as a sore that is not healing or is getting worse—is recommended.
- Yearly gynecology visits for women
- Evaluations of prostate health for men
- Dental care
  - ◆ Dentures can become loose with weight loss.
  - ◆ Untreated and undiagnosed dental pain can be the source of behavioral disturbances (crying, agitation), and possibly lead to more serious medical conditions such as infections.

What is complementary and alternative medicine (CAM)?

This term refers to nontraditional treatments and medications that people try in addition to, or instead of, those typically prescribed and recommended by Western physicians and other mainstream health care providers. With regards to Alzheimer's and other dementias there has been tremendous interest in various vitamins and herbal supplements—such as the antioxidants vitamins E and C and gingko biloba—as well as whether or not certain foods can prevent the onset of Alzheimer's or slow its progression.

In addition, there are various therapeutic techniques that have been tried to decrease the behavioral and emotional problems associated with dementia. These include music therapy, aromatherapy, massage, and other non-medication strategies that carry little risk and may have some benefit.

How should I decide whether or not to try different types of CAM?

When considering the use of complementary and alternative methods of treatment, the most import thing is to carefully weigh potential risks and benefits. If you are considering nutritional, herbal, or vitamin supplements, it's important to do so in communication with your prescribing physician or advanced practice nurse. There is a common myth that because something is "natural" it carries no risk of harm, side effects, or adverse reactions. This is not true. Plants and other natural substances are the basis of many potent and useful prescription medications—everything from aspirin to the heart medication digitalis to the blood-thinner coumadin. If taken incorrectly or in combination with the wrong other substances, natural supplements can be dangerous and even lethal.

Another important caution with herbal, nutritional, and vitamin supplements is that there is little regulation and standardization. Different companies prepare the substances in different ways, and in the United States it's difficult to know if you are getting the amount and type of the substance that has been studied and reported to be helpful.

What is ginkgo biloba?

Ginkgo biloba (also known as the maidenhair tree) is one of the most widely used over-the-counter preparations for its purported benefits to memory and mood. Extract of the ginkgo biloba tree leaf (EGb 761) has undergone a number of studies for dementia treatment, especially vascular dementia and Alzheimer's disease. The results have varied and it's not conclusive whether or not this is a useful substance. Many early studies of ginkgo showed promise for stabilization of memory loss and improvement in mood and functioning; however, this was not supported, or fully supported, by later, larger, and more carefully designed studies.

The typical dose of ginkgo (EGb 761) is 120 mg a day in divided doses, although some studies reported using doses of up to 240 mg per day. It is believed that at least four to six weeks of this regimen are required to evaluate whether or not it is of benefit. Ginkgo is generally well-tolerated, but there are cautions against combining it with blood thinners and antidepressants. Reported side effects include nausea, headache, and rash. Where ginkgo affects a part of the blood involved with forming clots (platelets) there is some concern that it may increase the risk of bleeding. As with any other medication, consult a doctor before taking and about the correct dosage.

What are antioxidants?

Antioxidants are certain vitamins (A, C, and E) and other substances that scavenge unstable charged particles (free radicals). Free radicals, because of their unstable nature—an unpaired electron—will bind with a stable molecule in an attempt to create a neutral charge. As they take the other molecule's electron, it in turn becomes a free radical. This process—oxidative stress or damage—is believed to be involved in a number of diseases, including Alzheimer's.

Based on this, it's been thought that using substances—antioxidants—that can bind free radicals and make them stable might be useful in the treatment of Alzheimer's. Numerous studies have been done looking at ascorbic acid (vitamin C), retinol (vitamin A), and tocopherol (vitamin E). While some studies have shown promise in delaying progression of Alzheimer's, the results are not robust or conclusive. Consult with your doctor or advanced practice nurse.

Does massage therapy help?

Massage therapy for a person with dementia can be a useful treatment, especially if it is something the person enjoys. Look for benefits such as an increased sense of well-being and calmness, as well as improved circulation and muscle-tone maintenance. Discuss this treatment with the person affected to see if it's something they will enjoy, or, if they have trouble communicating, consult their doctor or prescribing advanced practice nurse.

What is aromatherapy?

Aromatherapy uses intensely concentrated plant oils that release the smell of whatever plant substance they have been made from. Aromatherapy can be used on its own, or the oil can be incorporated into massage therapy. There are different ways people release the fragrance of the oils; you could put a few drops into an atomizer and spray it, or put a couple of drops into a bowl of heated water.

Studies looking at aromatherapy in dementia have found some small benefit in decreasing agitation. Oils that may be of particular benefit include melissa (lemon balm) and lavender. The only cautions would be that some people are disturbed by strong smells, and it's possible that a person could have an allergic reaction to a particular oil.

What is music therapy?

Music therapy uses music, singing, and often movement to help people communicate in ways other than speaking. It is provided by trained and certified therapists who assess how musical interventions may assist with someone's emotional and cognitive functions. It is more than just putting a CD on the stereo, and for people with dementia, and Alzheimer's in particular, it can be useful in a number of ways. Often a music-therapy session will involve using music and songs from the person's youth, which they may well remember. Along with the words and the melodies often come memories that are important to the person—their school years, dating, and so forth. Because different parts of the brain retain music, it's quite possible that even people who have severely limited speech and verbal recall are able to participate in, enjoy, and benefit from music therapy.

A number of studies have been done using music therapy with people who have Alzheimer's. Possible benefits include an enhanced sense of relaxation and well-being, improved sleep, and a decrease in behavioral problems.

What is reminiscence therapy?

Alzheimer's and most other dementing illnesses destroy memory in a backwards fashion—remembering what happened two minutes ago becomes impossible, but the name of your first-grade teacher may still be present, even into a moderate phase of dementia. Because old memories may still be present and accessible, reminiscence therapy can be an enjoyable activity for someone with dementia; it can comfort them and give them a feeling of control over their minds. Some researchers believe that accessing old memories may help to preserve them.

Reminiscence activities can involve:

- Going through an old photo album
- Picture books of activities the person used to enjoy, such as bowling or dancing
- Watching old television shows or movies that the person would have seen as a child or young adult
- Encouraging the person to recall important past events in their life
  - *"Tell me about the first time you met Grandma?"*
  - *"What was it like going to school in the '40s?"*

Encourage the person who is reminiscing to comment on whatever they are seeing and remembering. This can be a pleasurable and relaxed way to pass an hour for both the dementia patient and the caregiver.

What is art therapy?

Art therapy for people with dementia provides activities where the person is encouraged to select materials (paint, markers, fabric, clippings from magazines, etc.) and create art. For many, creating art is a calming process that also provides the person with a sense of accomplishment. At the end of the activity the person may be encouraged to talk about what they've made and why they selected particular materials, colors, or images.

If the person with dementia connects with the art therapy and enjoys it, having ready access to art supplies or craft materials can become a useful focus for their time and attention. These "busy boxes" can be kept in easy reach and provide a great deal of enjoyment, as well as comfort in times of distress or frustration. What goes in to a particular person's box will be based on their interests. For someone who likes to knit, sew, or crochet, the box could contain various yarns, ribbons, knitting needles, safety scissors, and patterns. For someone who likes to sketch, it could include paper, colored pencils, etc.

Can exercise prevent dementia or decrease its severity?

There is good evidence to support the long-held belief that maintaining a healthy body can both improve and sustain the brain's functioning. Studies comparing the rates of dementia in people who walk or exercise regularly and people who don't find decreased rates of dementia in the group that exercises. Other studies that have specifically focused on depression have also shown benefit for improving mood with regular exercise.

The type of exercise need not be strenuous, and walking is one of the most-studied forms. The exercise should be a part of the person's daily schedule, with at least thirty to forty-five minutes a day most days of the week.

Does drinking red wine prevent Alzheimer's?

There have been studies in France and New York looking at regular drinkers of moderate amounts of red wine (two to four standard glasses a day). These studies have both shown decreased rates of developing dementia in the wine drinkers.

It is not recommended, however, for people who already have dementia to be given any quantity of alcohol, as it will worsen confusion and may bring on unwanted behavioral outbursts. Additionally, it is not recommended for people to take up drinking wine in the pursuit of lowering their risk for developing dementia.

Chapter 7

Taking Care of the Whole Person

- How do I talk to Mom when she is confused?
- What is validation technique?
- What is therapeutic lying?
- Do people with dementia feel pain?
- How can I tell if my wife is in pain?
- What can I do to lessen my husband's physical pain?
- How can a social worker or case manager help me with my father?
- How do I get a social worker or case manager?
- What kinds of things can a visiting nurse do?
- What do home health aides provide?
- What services do occupational therapists (OTs) provide?
- How do I find an occupational therapist?
- What is adult day care?
- When should I consider enrolling my father in adult day care?
- How will I pay for adult day care?
- How important is exercise?
- How important is religion?

How do I talk to Mom when she is confused?

Joan felt her tension mount as her mother insisted, "You stole my pearls. You're taking all my things."

"No, mother," Joan said, for at least the eighth time since they'd gotten in the car. "Your pearls are in your jewelry box. You keep taking them out and hiding them."

"They are not! I would never do that. You stole my pearls."

When caring for someone with dementia, it's important to remember—and remind yourself again and again—that their brain no longer works as it once did. The usual give-and-take of conversation and of one person reasoning with another is disrupted. This becomes an important point because your loved one may still look the same and, on the surface, sound pretty logical. The next thing to keep in mind is that because the person with dementia is having problems with memory, this also means they will be unable to retain much, or any, new information. In other words, if you're trying to teach them something new—like where the mustard is kept—it will be hard for them to learn this, if not impossible.

This brings us to an important discussion on how you can learn to be as effective as possible in understanding and communicating with a person who has dementia. Because their ability to learn is seriously impaired, it is the caregiver that needs to find ways to get through the rough spots. For many, you will find yourself naturally slipping into different ways of talking with your loved one. In this and the following questions, we'll look at some specific strategies that might help. Here are some general techniques:

- Stay calm.
- Pay attention to the pitch of your voice and the emotion behind it. Your voice tends to rise in pitch and volume as you get upset. Try to deliberately keep your voice low, and try to speak in soothing tones.

- Don't insist on being right, even if the other person is dead wrong. Arguing with a person with dementia gets you nowhere.
- Once an argument develops, remind yourself that it's going to be pointless, and try shifting the conversation to something else; this is called a distraction technique. Or you could begin a new activity (let's fold clothes, watch TV, listen to music, go for a walk, etc.).

What is validation technique?

Frank listened as Carol, his wife, fretted about their daughter, "Alice has cancer. I just know it, the, doctor lies."

He knew that Alice was fine but lately Carol had gotten it into her head that their daughter was terminally ill, and nothing he could say would change her mind. He wondered if this didn't have to do with Carol's mother dying from cancer, and that she had lately started to confuse her daughter with her mother. Rather than once again try to correct his wife, which seemed to get her angry, he tried a different strategy. "You seem very upset," he said.

"I am. I'm very upset."

"I know," he said, "but we'll make it through this, and so will she. I promise."

"You promise."

"Yes dear, I promise."

Validation is a type of communication where we support a person's belief or feeling, no matter how outlandish it might be. Everyone likes to be validated; it makes us feel good, like getting a reward or an emotional pat on the back. In the case of someone with dementia, where they can so easily confuse and misinterpret situations, learning how to validate their world view and what they are experiencing—instead of constantly trying to correct them—can help them stay calm and decrease a typical source of stress between them and their caregiver(s).

It may take a bit of doing on your part to figure out how you can do this on a consistent basis. Practice helps. Some tips that can get you started include:

- When you find yourself getting set to argue with a person with dementia, catch yourself, stop, and ask:
    - Is this argument important?
    - Is there any chance I will win it?
    - Is it just going to make both of us more upset and stressed out?
    - Will they even remember it three minutes from now?
- See if you can find a way to take what the person is saying and support it, even if you don't fully agree—or agree at all.
    - *"You're so right, broccoli is nasty."*
    - *"Your pearls are missing? You always loved those pearls; why don't we go look for them later."*
- See if you can imagine what the person is saying as having a flow or direction—similar to approaches used in the martial art of aikido, where you take an opponent's attack and gently shift its direction.
    - A trip to the doctor: *"Yes, I know you don't like going to the doctor, Dad. I sure don't, let's go for a drive instead."* (And if you wind up at the doctor's afterward, so be it.)
    - Trouble in the shower: *"You are so right, the water is too cold. Let's warm it up. Tell me when you like the temperature. Is that good?"*

What is therapeutic lying?

Ivan hated the daily struggle of trying to get his mother dressed so he could take her to adult day care. The minute he mentioned this, she started to cry, and by the end they'd both be so upset that the entire morning was ruined. He noticed that at home his mother—who had been a wonderful seamstress and garment worker—liked to play with fabric, ribbon, and buttons. So one day when it was time to get her ready for day care, he came in with a basket of sewing notions and said, "Let's get dressed for work." There were no tears, and from then on he approached the daily dressing routine as "getting ready for work."

Therapeutic lying is another approach that can decrease the stress of caring for a person with dementia. It's a bit controversial, because most people believe in being scrupulously honest; the idea of lying, or deliberately misleading someone, can seem wrong. However, in the case of being a caregiver for a person with dementia, if used in the interest of helping or soothing them, white lies can be kind and humane.

There are two broad areas where you may find therapeutic lying to be useful:

1. Withholding information that the person might find upsetting, and that they won't remember anyway. This might even include the diagnosis of Alzheimer's or other dementing illness.

2. When the person with dementia misperceives something, rather than argue the point, just go along with it. This can include false beliefs that dead relatives are still alive, or that the person is still living in their own home, even if they are now in your home or a convalescent home. If the person is having persistent hallucinations (seeing things or hearing things that aren't there)—as can occur with some dementias—therapeutic lying means not trying to talk them out of it, but just letting them be, especially if they are not distressed by them.

Do people with dementia feel pain?

The ability of the body to feel pain and the body to perceive it is a primitive warning system that tells us something isn't right. Because people with moderate and more advanced forms of dementia cannot tell you that they are in pain, some professionals have theorized that advancing dementia brings the absence of pain; this is not true. People with dementia do feel pain, but because of their inability to communicate it or to remember it, the challenge for caregivers is to identify the source of pain and alleviate it.

How can I tell if my wife is in pain?

In the early stages of dementia, the person will probably be able to say that they are in pain, and to tell you what's hurting them. As short-term memory fails, it's likely that a pain that is only there with movement—such as arthritis pain, back pain, or pain on exertion as is seen with cardiac pain (angina)—may not be remembered when the person is sitting or lying still.

As verbal abilities decline, especially the ability to find the right words, people will not be clear about what hurts and where. It becomes increasingly important to look for physical and nonverbal cues. Is the person limping? Do they grimace and clamp their jaw when they try to get out of a chair? Do they sound like they are in pain when they go to the bathroom? When they try to chew? Alternatively, do they seem to suddenly be out of pain when they shift position or come to rest? Or are there new changes in behavior where they seem to cry or be much more agitated or irritable than is normal? Someone who suddenly refuses to eat or drink might be experiencing horrible dental pain. These kinds of clues will help lead you to the source of pain.

What can I do to lessen my husband's physical pain?

Depending on where the pain is coming from, the principles are basic: if possible, treat and eliminate the source of pain. This serves the double purpose of attending to a medical issue and making the person more comfortable. Things that fall in this range include infections (ear, urinary tract, painful boils, etc.), hemorrhoids, severe constipation, dental pain, cardiac pain/angina. If it's not possible to ease or eradicate the pain, as is the case with conditions such as arthritis that can cause chronic pain, work with your healthcare providers to decrease the pain.

Try giving the person pain medications prior to having them do something that you know may be painful, like taking a walk. If you use this strategy it will be important to give the medicine enough time to work. For chronic pain, such as arthritis, work with your physician or advanced practice nurse to find a daily regimen that will keep your loved one pain-free, or at the lowest level possible.

Other pain syndromes may be progressive and related to serious and even terminal conditions, such as invasive tumors and cancers. In these instances, aggressive use of narcotic pain relievers may be recommended. The downside here is that while you will decrease or eliminate pain, the level of confusion will go up.

Finally, some painful conditions come and go, such as hemorrhoids, angina, severe constipation, urinary tract infections, bed sores, dental pain, etc. You'll need to keep an eye out for these problems and get them attended to.

How can a social worker or case manager help me with my father?

Depending on your situation and the stage of dementia of the person you're caring for, social work and case-management services can assist you in a variety of ways. A case manager with experience working with dementia can provide education and identify various resources and agencies that can help you create a workable treatment plan. The case manager will help you identify what your current insurance will cover, and where you might be able to access low-cost, sliding-scale, or no-cost services. They will likely refer you to an attorney with expertise in elder law so that important legal and financial matters get addressed as soon as possible. They will also pay attention to the caregiver's level of stress and offer recommendations to help ease emotional distress. Some social workers may also be able to provide supportive therapy to the caregiver(s).

Case managers or social workers can help you think through important decisions, and in the later stages of the illness can assist with placement in an extended-care facility or convalescent home (see Chapter 15).

How do I get a social worker or case manager?

Social-work or case-management services can be obtained a number of different ways. Often, a case manager or social worker is a part of the dementia-assessment team. Some geriatric specialists will also have a case manager or social worker on staff. Community agencies that work with older people and their families will also use a case manager model.

Social-work services are available at hospitals. Should placement to a nursing home or extended-care facility be necessary, a social work consult will be obtained by the treating physician so that they can assist with the process of finding a suitable residential placement.

What kinds of things can a visiting nurse do?

Visiting nurses can provide a broad range of services, under a physician's written order. During the first visit, they will typically do an in-home assessment. This can be quite similar to what an occupational therapist does when they perform a home evaluation. The nurse will want to see how the person is able to get around the home, and what they are safely able to do in the bathroom, bedroom, and kitchen. Based on their findings and the person's medical and social needs, they will draw up a treatment plan that will include the kinds of services they will provide, how often they will be provided, as well as some services that could be done by paraprofessionals, such as home health aides or certified nurse's assistants (CNAs).

In addition, an in-home nurse can:

- Assess the person's overall level of wellness; if there are active, untreated medical problems they can alert the physician, or if necessary, contact emergency services to get the patient to a hospital.
- Assist with setting up and administering medications, including intravenous medications if necessary.
- Provide education to both the patient and the caregiver(s).
- Provide communication to the prescribing physician (the one who wrote the order for the in-home services), about how the person is progressing and what is being worked on in their treatment plan (plan of care).
- Provide dressing changes and ensure that any medical equipment is functioning.
- Recommend additional services, such as a home-health aide, physical or occupational therapist, social work assessment, etc.

There are stringent rules around what in-home nursing services Medicare and Medicaid will cover. While we will go into specifics in Chapters 11 and 12, in order to be eligible for reimbursement, all services provided must be deemed "medically necessary" and under a physician's order. Additionally, for Medicare to pay for the services, the person must be considered "homebound" (see Chapter 11).

What do home health aides provide?

Home health aides can assist with much of the day-to-day care of a person with dementia. They can help with basic tasks, such as cooking and cleaning, and while they cannot administer medications—physically give them to their patient—for legal reasons, in many instances they can oversee and direct the person to self-administer.

Areas where home health aides or certified nurse's assistants (CNAs) can be quite useful include:

- Bathing
- Light housekeeping, including laundry
- Preparing and serving meals
- Transportation (not always provided with some agencies; check before hiring, if this is a priority for you)
- Shopping
- Emotional support and company

A certain amount of home health aide services may be covered under Medicare and your state's Medicaid. If you have long-term health insurance this may be one of the covered benefits. These services can also be purchased through nursing agencies for as many, or as few, hours as desired. For families who have the financial resources to do so, an in-home, around-the-clock aide may be the best strategy for caring for their loved one with dementia.

What services do occupational therapists (OTs) provide?

Occupational therapists (OTs) provide some of the most useful assessments and strategies for working with people with dementia. OTs can work with individuals and their caregivers as part of an overall dementia evaluation, and they can also provide ongoing assessment and guidance in the home.

OT assessments are where the rubber meets the road for many people—they will help you and the person with dementia develop workable strategies using your/their own belongings and the layout of the home. Depending on the stage of the dementia, an OT will suggest different strategies for overcoming various problems. In early dementia, when it may still be possible for the person to function at their job, an occupational therapist might teach and supervise their patient using public transportation, instead of them driving to work. In the workplace, an OT will look at tasks that may be getting too difficult and see if there are ways to modify them so that the person can still function and meet the needs of the position. Where work is such an important function in terms of peoples' sense of purpose, financial well-being, independence, and meaning, being able to prolong an individual's work life may be an important goal.

As the dementia progress, OTs can be invaluable in figuring out what needs to be done in the bathroom and the kitchen to decrease the likelihood of falls and dangerous accidents. They will help you safety-proof the house as well as identify things you wouldn't be likely to think of, such as getting chairs that require the least amount of effort to get into and out of (likely, chairs that have higher seats than usual and have sturdy arms).

In later stages, problems with coordination, dressing, bathing, and eating will lead the OT to develop new solutions (see Chapter 10). The OT will work in coordination with your physician or treatment team; for instance, if specific pieces of medical equipment are needed—walkers, special raised toilet seats, wheelchairs, a riser chair, etc.—the OT will communicate this to your physician, who will write the actual order.

Basic principles that guide the OT include helping the person with dementia stay safe while preserving as much of their independence as is possible. The OT assesses what skills still remain and determines how to maximize these to get around areas of lost function.

How do I find an occupational therapist?

Depending on where you live, finding an OT—particularly one experienced in working with dementia—can be difficult. However, most geriatricians and other specialists who work with dementia will either have an OT working with them, as is sometimes seen in the larger dementia clinics, or they will be able to refer you to OTs they have worked with in the past.

Many in-home nursing agencies will also either employ a full-time OT or be able to access one on an as-needed basis. This is probably the best route to go, especially since in-home OT assessments are so useful. The OT assessment will need to be ordered by the physician or nurse practitioner that you are working with to be reimbursed by Medicare or other insurance; you may want to verify beforehand how much of the evaluation they will cover.

What is adult day care?

Adult day care centers provide socialization and structure for people with moderate and moderate-to-severe dementia. They are largely activity-based and might include crafts, reminiscence groups, singing, listening to music, movement, and gentle exercise and stretching. Many centers offer services seven days a week, and people can enroll for full-day and half-day sessions. Meals are typically included in the cost.

Adult day care can be a lifesaver for caregivers, providing respite as well as regular contact with people used to working with dementia who understand exactly what you're going through. Many adult day care centers offer additional services, including transportation and even showering and bathing.

When should I consider enrolling my father in adult day care?

The decision to use adult day care is one that should incorporate both you and the person you care for. Adult day care helps preserve social functioning by keeping people busy and occupied, and promotes general wellness through low-stress exercise and stretching. Various other activities, such as singing, movement, games, and music, access parts of the brain that may be less damaged by the dementing illness.

If you decide to use adult day care it's common for the person with dementia to not want to go, or to have a tough time adjusting. This usually passes, and the more you're able to build this into a part of a regular routine, the less disruptive it will be to your loved one.

For the caregiver, an adult day care center offers hours off to take care of yourself, other members of your family, and the day-to-day stuff that gets pushed aside when you're in the constant caregiver mode. Another benefit of adult day care is that it provides additional pairs of eyes that can help identify problems and problems in the making:

- *"I think she has a urinary tract infection."*
- *"He has a hard time hearing; should he get his ears checked?"*
- *"He's having trouble using his cane; is it time for a walker?"*

And for those centers that provide assistance with bathing and hygiene, this will be a welcome relief.

How will I pay for adult day care?

In Chapter 13 we will go over financial planning and how to access resources. Because adult day care is typically not covered by Medicare and other insurance, it may seem out of reach financially. Here are some suggestions that may help:

- Get a financial commitment from other family members. If split a number of ways, the financial burden may be manageable.
- Negotiate with the day care center. Ask if they have partial, or even full, scholarships. See if there is a price break if you provide your own transportation.
- Check with your state or local counsel or agency on aging (See Appendix D for a state-by-state listing) to see if there are grants or other forms of funding available for adult day care.
- In some states, adult day care may be covered under the Medicaid benefit.
- Check with your local Alzheimer's Association branch to see if they provide, or are aware of, any assistance for adult day care.
- If you have long-term health insurance, this may be a covered benefit.

How important is exercise?

The importance of daily exercise, including walking, cannot be stressed enough. Regular exercise is associated with:

- Better sleep and maintenance of sleep patterns
- Diminished levels of anxiety and depression
- Maintaining bone and muscle strength and health
- Helping maintain heart and lung function (circulation)
- Strengthening the immune system
- An overall sense of well-being

While some individuals with dementia will have physical disabilities that make regular exercise a challenge, most will not. Finding ways to include exercise in the daily schedule is important. Strategies might include:

- Taking daily walks with your loved one
- Signing up together to take a gentle yoga or stretching class

- Enrolling in an adult day care program that includes an exercise group
- Signing up for regular exercise groups at the local senior center
- For people in convalescent homes or extended care facilities (nursing homes), make sure that daily exercise is incorporated into the schedule.

How important is religion?

- *"Mom always went to mass. Now that she can't make it to church, I put it on the TV every morning at ten."*
- *"I know my husband doesn't remember much from the visits, but he seems to like having the rabbi visit."*

A person's religious beliefs, faith, and spiritual practices are highly individual and run the gamut from being immensely important and meaningful to inconsequential. For many, the rituals, practices, and beliefs of the religion in which they grew up, or which they adopted as adults, are a source of emotional strength and support.

Religious rituals, such as going to church/temple/mosque, are an important part of the weekly or daily routine for many people. Finding ways to maintain and even strengthen faith-based practices can help give a sense of normalcy and provide needed times for quiet and reflection for a person with dementia. Also, the hymns and prayers of their youth may be remembered well into the disease and give them a degree of comfort and pleasure.

When taking the person with dementia to religious services, sit near an exit in case the person becomes loud or agitated. You'll also want to attend a service that is less crowded, to try and decrease the overall level of stimulation.

Religious communities often offer an array of services—in addition to the religious and spiritual components—that can help ease caregiver burden. Many churches and temples will have friendly visitor programs, meal programs, senior programs, and possibly even transportation help.

Chapter 8 MEDICATIONS

- Are people with dementia at greater risk for side effects of medication?
- What can I do to decrease the risk of side effects and adverse reactions?
- Are there medications that can cure Alzheimer's?
- What can I expect from Alzheimer's medications?
- What are the cholinesterase inhibitors?
- What are the pros and cons of the different cholinesterase inhibitors?
- How can I combat the nausea from my cholinesterase inhibitor?
- If I get bad side effects with one cholinesterase inhibitor, should I try another?
- What is memantine (Namenda)?
- Is it okay to take both a cholinesterase inhibitor and memantine?
- What does it mean if a medication is being used "on label" or "off label"?
- When are tranquilizers and antipsychotic medications used?
- What are the side effects and adverse reactions of antipsychotic medications?
- When are antidepressants used?
- What are the different antidepressants that might be prescribed?
- How do I know if the antidepressant is working?
- Dad got put on an antidepressant; he's now agitated and can't sleep. What do I do?
- When are sleeping aids used?
- What are mood stabilizers and when are they used?
- How can I tell if a medication is working or not?

Are people with dementia at greater risk for side effects of medication?

For a number of reasons, the answer is yes. As we age, our bodies handle medications differently. The rate at which we eliminate (metabolize) different drugs slows down. This gets coupled with the fact that many older Americans will be taking multiple medications, which increases the risk for drug-to-drug interactions.

There are also a number of risks associated with the effects of medications on people with dementia:

- The accuracy with which someone with dementia will follow their prescription; they're at risk of taking too much or too little. *"I can't remember if I took it or not."*
- Extreme sensitivity to side effects, especially with medications that can increase symptoms of agitation and confusion.
- In moderate and advanced dementia, the person may be unable to communicate adverse reactions, such as constipation, urinary retention, or worsening confusion. If not carefully monitored by others, these seemingly small events could progress to a bowel obstruction, kidney damage, or a toxic delirium.

What can I do to decrease the risk of side effects and adverse reactions?

While perhaps obvious, the best way to avoid a side effect is to avoid a medication that might not be necessary. In dementia, especially when treating some of the behavioral symptoms—agitation, depression, hallucinations, delusions, anxiety, aggressiveness, sleep disturbances, etc.—it may be that we can avoid an additional pill through the use of nonmedication interventions (see chapters 9 and 10).

When medications are prescribed for people with dementia, doctors generally follow the golden rule of geriatric medicine: "start low and go slow." For family and caregivers, this means being on the lookout for new side effects and symptoms whenever a medication is added or there is a change in dose. Because of the way medications work in our bodies, side effects and adverse reactions may show up right away or could develop over days and weeks.

Things you can do to help decrease the risks include:

- Whenever a medication is changed or added, ask your doctor or pharmacist to run a drug-to-drug interaction profile. Most of them will have computer software that does this.
- Be sure that you or a family member always carries an updated list of all medications, including nutritional supplements and over-the-counter medications. Make sure that your physician and any other prescriber is aware of everything you are taking.
- If caring for someone with a moderate or greater degree of dementia, be on the lookout for any change—emotional, behavioral, or physical—whenever a medication is added or increased.
  - Are they more confused?
  - Are they complaining of stomach cramps, which might be a sign of severe constipation or urinary retention?
  - Are they less steady on their feet?
  - Do they become lightheaded when they shift positions?

Finally, each time you meet with the physician or advanced practice nurse, initiate a discussion on existing medications and dosages—is there something that could be safely lowered or stopped? It's frequently the case in older persons, especially those on complicated medication regimens, that it's not what you add, but what you reduce or take away, that will create the greatest improvement.

Are there medications that can cure Alzheimer's?

At present there are no known cures for Alzheimer's disease. However, there are medications that can moderately slow, but not reverse, the progression of this disorder. These are fully discussed in this chapter.

What can I expect from Alzheimer's medications?

Medications used to slow the progression of dementia can help decrease problem behaviors and improve overall functioning. They can help lengthen the time that a person will be able to stay in their own home before needing placement in a nursing home by as long as six to twelve months, as well as improve behavioral and emotional changes such as agitation, aggression, depression, and delusions. The medications do not change the course of the underlying disease—the damage in the brain—and will not prolong life, but they can help make life with dementia more comfortable and manageable.

For caregivers, these medications can make a real difference in the day-to-day experience of caring for someone with dementia. However, their benefits are usually modest at best, and so it's important to set realistic expectations.

What are the cholinesterase inhibitors?

The cholinesterase inhibitors are drugs that increase the amount of a naturally occurring chemical in the brain called acetylcholine. Acetylcholine acts as a chemical messenger between nerve cells (neurons); the cells destroyed by Alzheimer's are rich in it.

There are three cholinesterase inhibitors that are commonly prescribed:

- donepezil (Aricept)
- rivastigmine (Exelon)
- galantamine (Razadyne)

The first of these medications on the market was tacrine (Cognex). It is rarely used today on account of significant side effects, including upset stomach, nausea, and vomiting, and because it needs to be taken four times a day.

The theory behind these medications is simple: because Alzheimer's disease is associated with the destruction of brain cells rich in acetylcholine, increasing the amount of this chemical should improve symptoms. Multiple studies comparing these medications to placebo (a sugar pill) have shown that they do improve function and behavior in patients with mild-to-moderate Alzheimer's disease. Donepezil (Aricept) is presently the only cholinesterase inhibitor with FDA approval for the use in moderate-to-severe Alzheimer's.

What are the pros and cons of the different cholinesterase inhibitors?

Medication	How Taken	FDA Approval (Indication)	Common Side Effects
Donepezil (Aricept)	5 mg at bedtime for 4–6 weeks, and then may increase to 10 mg at bedtime.	Alzheimer's, mild to severe	nausea, vomiting, diarrhea, vivid dreams
Rivastigmine (Exelon, Exelon Patch)	1.5 mg twice a day for two weeks then increase slowly to a maximum of 12 mg per day.	Alzheimer's, mild to moderate; Parkinson's disease dementia, mild to moderate	nausea, vomiting, diarrhea
Galantamine (Razadyne, Razadyne ER)	8 mg daily in the morning for 4 weeks and then increase as tolerated to a maximum of 24 mg per day.	Alzheimer's, mild to moderate	nausea, vomiting, diarrhea

How can I combat the nausea from my cholinesterase inhibitor?

To decrease stomach upset when taking a cholinesterase inhibitor, don't take them on an empty stomach and start them at the lowest possible dose and increase gradually.

If I get bad side effects with one cholinesterase inhibitor, should I try another?

It is reasonable to try switching medications, if someone has intolerable side effects with one of these medications. Of the three, donepezil (Aricept) may have the lowest incidence of overall side effects; but, as with any medication, start slow and low.

What is memantine (Namenda)?

At present, memantine (Namenda) is the only other medication with FDA approval for the treatment of moderate to severe Alzheimer's disease. It works on a different chemical messenger in the brain than the cholinesterase inhibitors—glutamate. A recent study of its usefulness in less severe forms of dementia showed it to be mildly beneficial.

As with the cholinesterase inhibitors, memantine (Namenda) helps slow the progression of the symptoms. Common side effects include dizziness, confusion, sluggishness (lethargy), headaches, and constipation. This medication typically is started at 5 mg per day and is increased weekly to a maximum dose of 20 mg day (10 mg twice a day).

Is it okay to take both a cholinesterase inhibitor and memantine ?

Yes—combination therapy with a cholinesterase inhibitor and memantine (Namenda) is now included in both American and some, although not all, European practice guidelines for the treatment of Alzheimer's.

What does it mean if a medication is being used "on label" or "off label"?

"On label" means that a medication has received FDA approval, also called an indication, for a particular use. In the case of Alzheimer's, this includes the cholinesterase inhibitors and memantine (Namenda). In order to receive an on label indication, a medication must be shown to be more effective than a placebo (sugar pill). FDA approval in no way implies that the medication is better—or worse—than other medications used for the same condition(s) that are currently on the market.

"Off label" simply means that a medication has not received FDA approval for a particular use. In the treatment of dementia, especially the behavioral disturbances—aggression, agitation, depression, and anxiety—many medications have been tried and found to be of some benefit. They are used widely, and this practice is known as off label prescribing. Off label prescribing is perfectly legal, and many of these medications and their usefulness—or lack thereof—in the treatment of Alzheimer's and other dementias are areas of great interest and study.

When are tranquilizers and antipsychotic medications used?

In the past, it was common practice to use antipsychotic medications—also known as neuroleptics and tranquilizers—to treat the hallucinations and agitation that can be associated with dementia. Recently this practice has been called into question, with the discovery that the use of the newer antipsychotic medications (the atypical antipsychotics) carries an increased risk of death in people with dementia. The FDA has ruled that manufacturers of these medications must include a strong warning (black box warning) about this risk on all of their package inserts and advertising.

Atypical Antipsychotics

Compound/Generic Name	Trade Name (s)
Clozapine	Clozaril
Risperidone	Risperdal
Aripiprazole	Abilify
Ziprasidone	Geodon
Quetiapine	Seroquel
Olanzapine	Zyprexa

It is now believed that even the older medications (typical antipsychotics) in this class carry a similar risk. That said, in cases of disabling psychosis including hallucinations and/or delusions or severe agitation and aggressiveness, these medications in very low doses might be tried after other preventative strategies have not worked.

Typical Antipsychotics

Compound/Generic Name	Trade Name
Chlorpromazine	Thorazine
Haloperidol	Haldol
Trifluoperazine	Stelazine
Fluphenazine	Prolixin
Thiothixene	Navane
Loxapine	Loxitane
Molindone	Moban
Thioridazine	Mellaril (The trade name was discontinued due to cardiac concerns, while the generic is still available.)

What are the side effects and adverse reactions of antipsychotic medications?

Both the newer and older antipsychotic medications carry a heavy side-effect burden. If they are to be used, it is important to closely monitor the patient for any worsening of existing symptoms or development of new symptoms. Common side effects can include:

- Sedation
- Increased gait unsteadiness
- An increased risk for falls
- Parkinsonism. These medications can mimic—but not cause—most of the symptoms of Parkinson's disease. This can include the person taking small shuffling steps, having trouble turning around, diminished facial expressions, and limbs that feel stiff and slightly jerky. Parkinsonism, unlike Parkinson's disease, is reversible and should go away when the medication is stopped or the dosage lowered.
- Dry mouth
- Constipation
- Urinary retention
- Weight gain can be quite extreme, especially with the atypicals olanzapine (Zyprexa), clozapine (Clozaril), and quetiapine (Seroquel)
- Atypicals have also been associated with a "metabolic syndrome" that, in addition to weight gain, can increase the chance of diabetes and unhealthy elevations in cholesterol and other lipids.
- Movement abnormalities. This includes a potentially irreversible condition called tardive dyskinesia (TD), where the person, while awake, will have unintentional movements, most typically of the tongue, lips, and mouth. In more severe cases

this can progress to the entire body. Common symptoms of TD include the tongue thrusting in and out of the mouth and lip smacking.

When are antidepressants used?

Symptoms of clinical depression—loss of energy, sadness, loss of interest, disturbed sleep and appetite, irritability, thoughts of death, feelings of hopelessness, etc.—are common in dementia. Because depression can be successfully treated with medication, it is quite common for an antidepressant to be recommended, as well as other nonmedication strategies, such as increasing activity level, exercise, and socialization.

What are the different antidepressants that might be prescribed?

At present there are a large number of antidepressant medications on the market. These include some of the most-widely prescribed medications in America. Here, antidepressants are broken into groups based on how they work on the brain.

Medications known as SSRIs (selective serotonin reuptake inhibitors) and SNRIs (selective serotonin and norepinephrine reuptake inhibitors) are typically the first antidepressants a doctor will try with a patient. These medications increase the relative amounts of serotonin (and norepinepherine, in some cases) available to the brain. It is believed that increases in these chemical messengers help in decreasing symptoms of depression, although the exact mechanism by which this happens is not fully understood. As there are several of these, it is reasonable to switch from one to another if there is no response or if the person has intolerable side effects.

Selective Serotonin Reuptake Inhibitors

Compound Name	Trade Name	Typical Dose Range
Citalopram	Celexa	10–60 mg/day
Escitalopram	Lexapro	10–20 mg/day
Fluoxetine	Prozac	10–60 mg/day
Paroxetine	Paxil	10–60 mg/day
Sertraline	Zoloft	50–200 mg/day

As with all antidepressants, SSRIs should be started at the lowest dose possible. As the SSRIs can cause a large number of drug-to-drug interactions, it is important to watch for any behavioral or physical changes. For people who are on medications that need to be maintained within specific limits, such as the blood thinner warfarin (Coumadin) or the anticonvulsant phenytoin (Dilantin), it will be important to check medication levels, or other blood tests, more frequently when an SSRI is being added or changed. In addition to drug-to-drug interactions, some of the SSRIs can also interact with certain foods, such as grapefruit juice, resulting in unwanted increases in drug levels.

Another class of antidepressants that may be tried includes ones that act on both serotonin and norepinephrine, sometimes referred to as SNRIs (selective serotonin and norepinephrine reuptake inhibitors). These include:

Selective Serotonin and Norepinephrine Reuptake Inhibitors

Compound/ Generic Name	Trade Name	Dose Range
Venlafaxine	Effexor, Effexor XR	75–375 mg/day
Duloxetine	Cymbalta	20–60 mg/day
Nefazodone	Serzone	300–600 mg/day Only available as a generic. The name brand was withdrawn from the market by the manufacturer on account of a few reports of liver toxicity, including liver failure.

Other antidepressants that may be prescribed include:

Compound Name	Trade Name	Dose Range	Comments
Buproprion	Wellbutrin, Wellbutrin XR, Zyban	150–450 mg/day	Unique; affects dopamine. Also used in smoking cessation. Associated with seizures in higher doses.
Mirtazipine	Remeron	15–45 mg, given at bedtime	Sedating and associated with weight gain
Trazodone	Desyrel	25–400 mg/day	Highly sedating, often used as a sleep aid. Men need to be cautioned about serious erectile adverse reaction (priapism).

Finally, there are two groups of older antidepressants that are less commonly prescribed—largely on account of a heavy side-effect burden. These include the tricyclic antidepressants (so called because of the way their molecular structure looks), and the monoamine oxidase inhibitors (MAOIs). MAOI users are required to strictly adhere to a diet free from a compound called tyramine, which is found in certain fruits, aged cheeses, alcohol, and more.

How do I know if the antidepressant is working?

There are a couple of important things to keep in mind when a person is taking antidepressant medication. First, they don't work right away, although you may experience side effects immediately. In general, you should not expect to see much benefit from an antidepressant for at least two to four weeks, often longer in older persons where the medication may need to be started at a lower-than-adequate dose to decrease the risk of unwanted side effects or drug interactions.

Once a person has been on the medication for a long enough time, and at an adequate dose, the best way to assess whether the medication is helping is by following the target symptoms of depression. These will vary from person to person, but may include:

- Are they less sad? Less withdrawn?
- Has their appetite improved?
- Has sleep improved?
- Do they appear more positive and hopeful?
- Are they less anxious?
- Are they more active and interested in things and people around them?
- Are they less focused on physical complaints and pains?
- Are they less focused on death?

Dad got put on an antidepressant; he's now agitated and can't sleep. What do I do?

When starting an antidepressant, or even when a person has been on one for a while, it's possible for the medication to bring on a more agitated state. This is especially true for people who have a history of bipolar disorder—antidepressant medications, especially when used without something to help keep the mood stable, can trigger a manic episode (a mood state where the person is more energized, or agitated, may speak rapidly, have unrealistic, often very grand thoughts, and gets little to no sleep).

Should this occur, it will be important to immediately contact your prescribing physician or advanced practice nurse. If the person is so agitated that you are concerned about their or your safety, they need professional help immediately. Depending on the medication and the person's overall medical and psychiatric condition, the doctor's recommendations will vary. Some medications can be discontinued immediately and the agitation should go away within a few days, while other medications might require tapering and/or a more monitored setting, such as a hospital stay.

When are sleeping aids used?

Disruption in sleep patterns is common in dementia. Middle of the night wandering, diminished sleep, and day-time napping may become so distracting that medication is recommended to help control them. However, prior to turning to medication there are a number of effective nonmedication strategies that can improve sleep; these are outlined on page 116.

The most important thing to keep in mind when trying a drug for sleep is if it's helping, or if it's just making the person more confused, unsteady on their feet, or agitated. Because people with dementia can be very sensitive to medications, and particularly to sedating ones, using the lowest effective dose is important.

You should also consider any drug interactions—if the person is already taking sedating medications, combining them with a sleep aid can greatly increase confusion, agitation, and unsteadiness. Also, many sleeping aids can cause physical dependence. If a person is taking them on a nightly basis, they should not be stopped abruptly. To avoid what could be a dangerous withdrawal, the person should have the medication tapered off.

Sleep aids that might be recommended by your physician or APRN include:

- Benzodiazepines—this is a group of drugs that include lorazepam (Ativan), clonazepam (Klonopin), temazepam (Restoril), diazepam (Valium), alprazolam (Xanax), and others. These are probably best avoided as they can worsen forgetfulness and confusion. If used, these should be tried in the lowest dose possible. Risks include dependency and an increased risk of falls because of their sedating quality.

- Diphenhydramine (Benadryl)—This over-the-counter antihistamine is one of the most widely-used sleep aids, and is probably best avoided in Alzheimer's as it may worsen confusion and unsteadiness. It is typically not considered habit-forming, but it does interact with many other medications. Other side effects can include constipation and urinary retention. Benadryl should not be used in people with certain types of glaucoma.

- Eszopiclone (Lunesta)—A typical dose is 1–2 mg in older persons. May cause dependence, and should not be taken immediately after eating a high-fat meal.

- Ramelteon (Rozerem)—A relatively new sleep aid that is taken nightly. The typical dose is 8 mg. May cause physical dependence, and should not be taken immediately after eating a high-fat meal.

- Trazodone (Desyrel)—This is an older antidepressant that is highly sedating. In low doses (25–100 mg) it can be an effective sleep aid. In men, trazodone carries a rare risk for a sustained painful erection (priapism), which requires urgent medical care.

- Zaleplon (Sonata)—Risks include increased confusion, agitation, and falls.

- Zolpidem (Ambien)—Potential risks with this drug include increased confusion and even some reported cases of delusions and/or hallucinations. Zolpidem has a short length of action and some people find that it helps them get to sleep, but then they wake up four hours later. There is also a longer-acting form of this medication.

What are mood stabilizers and when are they used?

Mood-stabilizing medications are most often associated with bipolar disorder. While the exact mechanisms by which these medications work are not fully known, they help to decrease the severity and frequency of both episodes of depression and mania. They include: lithium, valproic acid (Depakote), and lamotrigine (Lamictal). While none of them are FDA-approved for use in the behavioral disturbances associated with dementia, it is sometimes appropriate to use medications such as valproic acid (Depakote) in low doses, to see if it decreases the overall level of agitation and combativeness. For some patients with severe agitation, who may not be able to tolerate some of the other medications, the mildly tranquilizing properties of these medications can at times help.

How can I tell if a medication is working or not?

The best way to assess any medication is to be clear why you or your loved one is taking it and whether that symptom has gotten better, worse, or stayed the same. If you have pain and you take a painkiller, does the pain go away? If a person's blood pressure is high, does it come down when the medication is used?

While simple in theory, seeing the effects of a medication becomes complicated when working with someone with significant dementia, as they may be unable to tell you if their pain or nausea has gone away. You, in conjunction with your medical professionals, will have to rely on the power of observation—what you see, smell, hear, and feel—and measuring through tests (such as checking blood sugar levels in a person with diabetes) those things that can be measured.

When using medication to improve behavioral problems such as crying, aggression, sundowning (a condition where the person becomes agitated and more confused in the late afternoon and evening), and catastrophic reactions, it's a good idea to keep track of:

- How often the behavior occurred before and after the medication was started.
- If the behavior still occurs, is it worse, better, or unchanged?
- Have new problems emerged since starting the medication? Does the person appear more or less confused?

If you're someone who likes to put things in writing, keeping a notebook or logbook where you jot down the frequency and severity of target symptoms may help you—and your treatment team—get a more objective view of whether or not different interventions have been effective.

Chapter 9

EMOTIONAL AND BEHAVIORAL CHANGES

- Why does my father become so upset so easily?
- How do I figure out what triggered the problem behavior?
- What can I do to decrease episodes of agitation?
- How can I stop my father from telling the same story over and over?
- How do I manage tantrums when I need to give my wife a shower?
- What can I do to get my husband to eat?
- How do I handle toileting?
- What is "sundowning"?
- How can I decrease my wife's agitation in the evening?
- How can I get my husband to sleep?
- How do I handle paranoia and accusations of stealing?
- My mother is seeing and hearing things; what should I do?
- Why is there so much depression associated with dementia?
- Is medication the only answer for the depression that can occur with dementia?
- Are people with Alzheimer's and dementia at increased risk for suicide?
- My husband says he wants to kill himself—how do I handle this?
- What do I do when my husband becomes abusive and tries to hit me?
- How can I help alleviate my wife's depression about being in a nursing home?
- The home sent my dad to the ER because he struck an aide; what do I do?
- What is normal sexual behavior in a person with dementia?
- Why has my father started exposing himself to others?
- How do I handle sexually inappropriate behavior?

Why does my father become so upset so easily?

"The littlest thing seems to set him off. It's not like him to get so upset."

It's difficult to predict the types of emotional and behavioral changes that come with dementia. Some individuals will continue to have bright and pleasant personalities even into the later stages. For others, the emotional upheavals and day-to-day tantrums (often referred to as catastrophic reactions) can be extreme and exhausting for caregivers. Catastrophic reactions can burn out caregivers and are often the deciding factor about whether or not to place someone in a long-term care facility. In this chapter we'll look at various types of emotional disturbances and present approaches that can help you through them.

A good place to begin thinking about this is by trying to put yourself in the place of your loved one. People with dementia are faced with a world of tasks that they are no longer able to do as well as they once could, or at all. Common emotional responses to this are frustration, anger, fear, anxiety, and depression. These emotional states then get paired with behaviors—it is the emotion, which can change rapidly and in response to something that seems trivial, that triggers what may be a catastrophic response.

Common pairings of emotions with behaviors are:

- Frustration and anger can lead to shouting, lashing out physically, and, in extreme cases, assaultiveness.
  - *"I told him he couldn't have a cigarette and he started to scream at me."*
  - *"He couldn't find the bathroom and accused me of having moved it."*
- Fear and anxiety can make the person withdraw from others, cry, and refuse to do whatever is being asked of them.
  - *"When I try to give Mom her bath, she refuses; the more I insist the worse it gets. She starts crying and telling me that I'm hurting her; it's horrible."*

- Depression leads to withdrawal and an overall diminished state of activity. The person may refuse to eat and to get out of bed. They may talk about wanting to die, and how much of a burden they have become.
- Boredom and loneliness can lead to pacing, rocking, and wandering.

How do I figure out what triggered the problem behavior?

In the previous question we looked at how emotions precede problem behavior. Let's take this a step further and see if we can identify what triggered the emotional response that led to the problem behavior. This approach of identifying triggers and the corresponding emotions and behaviors is the basis of cognitive-behavioral therapy, which is used with depression and anxiety and is also useful in working with people with dementia. It's a strategy that, if practiced, will give you a way to think through difficult scenarios and help you find solutions.

Trigger	Emotional Response	Problem Behavior
"I can't give you a cigarette now."	Frustration and anger	Screams and paces back and forth

Triggers take many forms, and as the person with dementia loses more of their verbal abilities it may become hard to know what might be setting them off.

- Could they be in pain: do they have severe constipation and cramping, is there a urinary tract infection brewing, could they have a bed sore?
- The trigger could be an unfamiliar setting or person, such as a new nursing home, day care center, or staff member.

- Problems in the physical environment—too noisy, too hot, too cold—could also trigger a catastrophic behavioral response.
- Being confronted with tasks that are too hard for them can generate frustration and fear.

Trigger	Emotional Response	Problem Behavior
Stomach cramps and physical pain	Depression and fear	Refusal to eat, screaming, rocking

What can I do to decrease episodes of agitation?

Once you have identified what is triggering an emotional and behavioral response, it's now a question of finding things you can do to eliminate or lessen the trigger. If you believe the person is in pain and this is fueling their nonstop screaming, try to address the source of pain. If the person appears frightened and is crying, seek out the source of their fear—whether real or imagined—and see if it can be eliminated. Alternatively, you might find that strategies such as distraction—let's go for a walk, feed the dog, listen to music—may put an end to the outburst, or prevent the outburst from occurring at all. Many find that gentle physical contact, even just a touch on the hand or shoulder, can be a useful tool for helping calm fears and quiet agitation.

Trigger	Emotion	Problem Behavior	Trigger Reduction
A trip to the doctor, "We have to see Dr. Jones."	Anger and rage	Refusal to get into the car, shouting	Distract with a snack, let a few minutes pass and then say, "let's go for a ride."

There will be a lot of trial and error that goes into figuring out what might be triggering a behavioral response, and the best way to soften it. Be creative, stay calm, and ask others what's worked for them; with practice you'll able to lessen the frequency and severity of outbursts.

How can I stop my father from telling the same story over and over?

People with dementia, especially in the early stages, will frequently tell the same story repeatedly. The stories typically involve important or meaningful events that happened earlier in their lives, and they will tell it as though it's for the first time. The best response is to listen politely, acknowledge the importance of the story, and then try to shift to another topic. There is no point in telling the person, "I've heard this story forty times." They don't remember that they told you. Getting upset or annoyed will likely only get them upset and annoyed.

How do I manage tantrums when I need to give my wife a shower?

Bathing and showering can become fraught with anxiety and fear in people with moderate and advanced dementia. The trigger to this emotional and behavioral outburst could be many different things or a combination of things—fear of water, fear of slipping and falling, fear of getting scalded, embarrassment over being naked in front of someone else, anger over loss of privacy, fear of being assaulted. So without knowing the specific trigger it's useful to think about all the kinds of things you can do to try to make the experience a pleasurable one—for both of you.

- Consider putting soothing music on in the background.
- Use soaps and products that they like and are familiar with.
- Make sure the bathroom is well-lit and warm. Let them keep their glasses on.

- Let them feel the water temperature before getting in.
- Make sure you have grab bars, and possibly a bath/shower seat so that they can feel more secure.
- Some people find that a handheld shower attachment may be easier, or less frightening to a person with dementia, than over-head shower heads.
- Stay calm. Don't let your voice get raised, regardless of how frustrated you may feel.
- Use humor and affection throughout the process—this doesn't mean you're cracking jokes, but it's good to smile and use facial expressions that let the person know you care and that they're okay.
- If the person had a previous bath or shower schedule, try to stick to it. If they only bathed every other day, don't insist on daily baths. If they always used a tub, consider that instead of a shower.
- Consider using other alternative forms of bathing, such as heated hygienic disposable bathing systems (Bag Bath).
- If modesty is an issue for the person with dementia, consider letting them bathe while wrapped in a bath sheet.

What can I do to get my husband to eat?

People with moderate and more advanced dementia will begin to experience problems at meal times. They might appear to have no appetite, get frustrated with accidents and spills, or be unable to handle a fork or other utensils. Adapting to these changes takes some trial and error. One way to think about this is that the person with dementia is going backwards through the various stages of learning. As a child first learns to use a bottle, then their hands, then a cup, and then cutlery, the person with dementia will be going in the opposite direction.

Healthy finger foods that the person can easily manage are one solution. Depending on the person's ability to chew and swallow, this could be anything from carrot and celery sticks, to chicken strips, granola bars, and other more easily managed foods. Leaving a bowl of a healthful snack in easy reach of the person may also ensure that they are getting adequate food. Spill-proof cups with a built-in straw are a good way to cut down on frustration and accidents.

If the person wants to keep using cutlery but is having difficulty, there are a couple of things that will help. Remember that every step you eliminate from a complex task makes it that much easier. Cut the food into bite-size pieces—this eliminates the need to coordinate a knife. If the person is struggling with the fork, sometimes taking their hand and starting the process will trigger the brain to remember that the fork needs to go from the plate to the mouth and back again.

For many people, meal times have always been a social event. What sometimes happens in nursing homes is that the meal is left with the person in their room and they don't eat it. The best way around this is to sit with the person—or have someone else sit with them—during mealtime and assist them as needed.

How do I handle toileting?

There are two guiding principles with toileting: You want to preserve the person's dignity while simultaneously ensuring good hygiene and health. Depending on the person's level of functioning, you will need to provide the appropriate level of support and oversight. However, because learning how to use the toilet is something we acquire as young children, for many with dementia the ability to use the bathroom persists even up through moderate and severe degrees of illness.

In the home, reminders about going to the bathroom—both physical and verbal—may be helpful. A sign on the bathroom door, or better yet, leaving the door open and a light on, may give the person important cues. If possible, you might want to arrange the bedroom so the person can see the bathroom from their bed; this will help decrease confusion should they need to use it in the night. Gentle reminders about going to the bathroom before bed and at other times throughout the day may also be effective. Also remember that as we get older our bladders lose some of their elasticity and so the need to urinate more frequently is common.

Adult protective underwear (Depends, Poise, etc.) will also decrease the likelihood of embarrassing accidents. Giving verbal or written reminders to wipe and wash hands will likely be necessary. Adult disposable wipes, marketed under various brand names, can also be used to enhance hygiene.

In advanced stages of dementia, where more hands-on assistance is required, additional concerns will include being alert for the development of sores and/or rashes in the buttocks and genital areas. Overall, a calm and gentle approach to toileting is the way to go. While we are talking about adults, there are a lot of parallels with the process of toileting and diapering an infant. Their health and safety is always a primary concern.

What is "sundowning"?

Sundowning describes increased levels of agitation and confusion in the late afternoon and evening. Typical behaviors may include shouting, wandering, or increased expressions of fear, sadness, and anxiety. Sundowning is common in dementia, and its causes are not entirely clear. It may have to do with the decreased levels of light worsening feelings of confusion. It may also have to do with disruptions in the normal sleep-wake cycle and the body's natural, circadian rhythms.

How can I decrease my wife's agitation in the evening?

There are a number of strategies you can try to decrease sundowning agitation. As with all interventions, not everything will work for everyone, or in every situation. You'll need to experiment a bit to see what helps in your situation. Some strategies that others have found useful include:

- Make sure the environment is well-lit. Some professionals theorize that decreased light and increased shadows may worsen confusion and disorientation.
- Ensure that the person gets adequate exercise and activity earlier in the day. This will make them tired in the evening and help regulate their sleep-wake cycle. If they're living in a nursing home, be sure that regular physical activity—if they are able—is included as part of their daily care plan.
- Be careful of foods and beverages that might worsen agitation, such as caffeinated beverages or caffeine-containing foods, like chocolate.
- Review with your healthcare provider if any of the medications your loved one is taking could be worsening confusion in the evening. If this is the case, ask if they can change the medications or shift dosing to an earlier time of day.
- Try playing soft music in the evening or late afternoon.
- Some find that leaving a television set playing can help orient the person.
- Make sure the bathroom is highly visible. Consider leaving the door open at all times.
- Ask your prescribing physician or APRN if there are any medication strategies that might decrease evening agitation. This strategy should only be tried once non-medication interventions have been exhausted.

How can I get my husband to sleep?

Disruption of a regular sleep-wake cycle and insomnia are common problems in dementia, and can be a source of considerable stress if the person is up at night wandering around the house. However, there are many things you can do to maintain or reestablish a more normal sleep pattern:

- Provide adequate daytime exercise and activity. Numerous studies have found benefits in daily exercise for promoting good sleep; this includes less strenuous forms of activity, such as walking.
- Discourage daytime naps.
- Establish and stick to a regular bedtime and a regular wake-up time.
- Eliminate caffeine from the diet.
- Make sure that the person's bed and sleeping environment are comfortable. This includes a good mattress and pillow and a room that is kept at a temperature the person likes and that is free from outside noises. If they would rather fall asleep in a chair in front of the television, that's okay.
- Consider a medical evaluation to look for other causes of insomnia, including sleep apnea (periods in the night where a person stops breathing).
- Reserve the bed for sleeping. Discourage the person from staying in bed during the daytime.

If the preceding doesn't work, consult with your prescribing physician or nurse practitioner about the use of sleep aids—these are discussed in Chapter 8. It's important to remember that sleeping medications all carry a risk of side effects and adverse reactions, such as an increased risk of falls and worsening of confusion, and many are habit-forming. If sleeping medication is to be used, it should be at the lowest effective dose, and preferably on an as-needed basis vs. a nightly dose.

How do I handle paranoia and accusations of stealing?

The paranoia (fear that people are out to hurt you) that frequently accompanies dementia is different than the paranoia we see in psychiatric disorders, such as schizophrenia. A person with dementia will go looking for something, not be able to find it, and then accuse people of having stolen it. *"You took my mother's jewelry." "She keeps stealing my glasses."*

Many families will also describe how the person with dementia may begin to hide things, forget where they hid them, and then accuse others of having taken them. Intellectually, we can see how this all stems from the loss of memory, but it can be very disturbing, embarrassing, and painful to have your mother accuse you of having robbed her blind in the middle of a grocery store.

The kinds of strategies that can diffuse this paranoia, at least for the moment, include simply reassuring the person that their jewelry is safe, their glasses are around their neck, or that you'll look for the missing item as soon as you can. Alternatively, you might try to gently shift them to a more pleasant topic.

My mother is seeing and hearing things; what should I do?

Visual and auditory hallucinations can be either a symptom of the dementia, such as is common in Lewy body dementia, or may be a sign of delirium. Delirium, a fluctuating level of alertness that is discussed in Chapter 3, will require prompt medical attention to determine the cause. However, if the hallucinations are a part of the dementia, the questions that need to be asked are:

- Is the person bothered by the hallucination?
- Do the hallucinations further limit the person's ability to function?
  - ◆ *"The green men won't let me get out of bed."*
  - ◆ *"Mother told me that you poisoned my food. I'm not eating."*
- Are they doing things in response to the hallucinations (command hallucinations)?
  - ◆ *"The voice told me to hurt myself."*

If the person is not bothered by the hallucinations, the best solution will be to do nothing. There's no point in arguing about whether or not there is a little girl in a red dress under the table. Because antipsychotic medications (discussed in Chapter 8) carry a high risk of side effects and adverse reactions, these should only be used—and in the lowest dose possible—when the hallucinations cause distress or significant functional impairment.

Why is there so much depression associated with dementia?

"Mom used to be so filled with life and now all she does is sit in her chair for hours. I can't get her to do anything. If I don't sit with her, she won't eat. Even when I bring the kids over she doesn't smile, and lately she's started saying, 'just let me die.' This just isn't like her."

Sustained episodes of depression are extremely common in all stages of dementia. It is estimated that roughly 50 percent of people with Alzheimer's will have symptoms of depression two years prior to being diagnosed. As the dementia progresses, researchers report levels of depression from mild to severe at around 40 percent. So not only is depression common with dementia, it is also a symptom that can occur before noticeable memory loss or other signs of impairment have developed.

The depression that occurs with dementia comes from a number of sources. It could be situational, such as grief over the loss of independence and functioning and/or unhappiness over being placed in a nursing home. In addition, a significant amount of depression is believed to be biologically triggered. Depression appears to be a natural response to a damaged brain, with increased levels of depression being common following strokes, and in the nerve damage seen in Alzheimer's disease, Parkinson's, and other neurologic disorders. Also, the risk for depression in dementia is higher for people who have experienced episodes of depression earlier in their lives.

Common symptoms of depression in people with dementia include:

- A sad or depressed mood
- Frequent tearfulness
- Changes in energy level, where the person either becomes inactive or seems agitated and always nervous
- Loss of appetite
- Changes in sleep, where the person either wants to spend the entire day in bed, or is unable to sleep
- Expressions of being worthless or beyond hope:
  - *"I'm such a burden."*
  - *"You'd all be better off without me."*
  - *"My life is over."*
- Thoughts or actions that indicate the person wants to die or is considering suicide:
  - *"I wish I were dead."*
  - *"I wish God would just take me."*
  - *"If I had a gun I'd shoot myself."*

Is medication the only answer for the depression that can occur with dementia?

No; and while there are few studies specifically targeting non-medication strategies with people who have both dementia and depression, the following list are things known to decrease levels of depression in general. As with most other forms of treatment with dementia, it's a process of trial and error—experiment until you determine what helps.

- Exercise—this can take the form of daily walking and gentle stretching. Studies comparing regular exercise to antidepressants in an older population found exercise to be of significant benefit, if it's at least thirty to forty-five minutes a day on most days of the week.
- Socialization and activity—many people with dementia struggle with intense loneliness. They have difficulty remembering that you were just there to visit. Keeping them active with a regular schedule will help combat depression. When choosing a convalescent home it will be important that they have adequate daily programming and activities.
- Regular routines—we are creatures of habit, and having a predictable schedule that includes a range of activities, socialization, regular meal times, bedtime, bath time, and wake-up time helps diminish anxiety and provides a sense of normalcy.
- Sunlight—daily exposure to sunlight or full-spectrum light.
- Physical contact, gentle touch, and massage.

Are people with Alzheimer's and dementia at increased risk for suicide?

It is well-documented that the group at highest risk for suicide in the United States is older white men. Since Alzheimer's and dementia are illnesses more associated with older people, this raises the question of whether or not this group is also at a higher risk for suicide. In general, the answer is no. However, suicidal statements, suicide attempts, and completed suicide can and do occur in this group. Be particularly aware of this if you're caring for someone who has previously attempted suicide, has a history of mental illness, and has access to lethal means of self-injury, such as firearms—the number one means of fatal suicide in this country. Also, people with dementia who attempt suicide are generally in the earlier stages of the illness, when they have a greater understanding of the illness and their prognosis and have a greater ability to plan and carry out a suicide attempt.

The wish to die has been reported in about 4 percent of people with dementia attending memory loss clinics. This number is much higher when caregivers are asked if their loved one has ever expressed a wish to die.

My husband says he wants to kill himself—how do I handle this?

Any suicidal statement or gesture must be taken seriously. The adage, "people who talk about killing themselves don't actually do it," is false. The majority of people who end up taking their own life have in fact discussed their feelings with family, friends, or a medical provider in the weeks and months before committing suicide. Another chilling fact is that the single highest risk group for committing suicide is older, white men, especially after a loss or diagnosis of illness. Do not assume that just because someone has dementia, especially in the earlier stages, they are unable to kill themselves.

If your loved one is talking about suicide or has made a suicide attempt (swallowed pills, tried to hang or drown themselves, made threatening gestures with a knife or firearm), get immediate help. This can be done by calling 911, or if your region has a mobile crisis unit, ask them to come out and assess the situation.

It is important that guns and other lethal means for suicide—such as medications, gas stoves, automobiles, etc.—are kept out of harm's way and are not accessible. If the person has made impulsive gestures, such as trying to jump from a moving car, walking into traffic, etc., seek help immediately.

What do I do when my husband becomes abusive and tries to hit me?

Lashing out physically is one of the behavioral problems that often results in placing someone into an extended-care facility, such as a nursing home. As with other negative behaviors, this is best approached with a calm, gentle, and non-confrontational manner. Admittedly, this is easier said than done when a person with dementia is having a catastrophic response and is behaving in a violent manner. While on one hand it may look much like a child's temper tantrum, the important difference is you're dealing with an adult who may have considerable physical strength. Our natural response when facing a threat—such as someone coming at us with a weapon or closed fist—is to fight back or get out of the way; this is an important survival mechanism. The first thing you must do is to consider your own safety. If someone is throwing things or coming at you as though they intend to strike you, get out of the way.

Next, if the situation cannot be quickly handled, or you feel that the person may harm you or someone else, do not hesitate to call 911 and get assistance. People with dementia can, and do, cause physical injury to others—most frequently their caregiver.

If the situation is less critical and you believe it can be safely handled, the previous approach of identifying triggering events, emotions, and behaviors may help you come up with solutions that can decrease the frequency of these outbursts. Ask yourself the question, "What got her so upset?" (the triggering event):

- Is she hungry?
- Is she in pain?
- Is there something in the house that upset her?
- Did I just ask him to do something he found frustrating?
- Is he depressed?

Once you think you've hit upon the triggering event, the next step will be to try and eliminate or decrease it. If they're hungry, get them a snack; try to locate the source of pain; simplify a task they found too difficult, etc.

Finally, in Chapter 8 we discussed medications. One of the findings with cholinesterase inhibitors donepezil (Aricept), rivastigmine (Exelon), and galantamine (Razadyne), as well as memantine (Namenda) and possibly some other drugs, is that they can decrease the overall frequency and severity of behavioral episodes—especially in the home.

How can I help alleviate my wife's depression about being in a nursing home?

A move into a nursing home can be traumatic for both the person with dementia and their caregiver(s). Most people, if given the choice, would prefer to remain in their own home. As we'll see, for many reasons— often related to behaviors discussed in this chapter—this may become no longer possible, and a nursing-home placement is necessary.

A typical emotional/behavioral response to being placed in a nursing home is depression, with episodes of tearfulness, a loss of appetite, anxiety, sadness, etc. Here, you've got a pretty good idea what the triggering event has been; now it's a question of what you can do to help the person settle more happily into their new surroundings.

Important things that may help include:

- Frequent and regular visits
- Photographs of family, pets, etc.

- A few personal belongings that can make their space appear more familiar, such as a quilt and some pillows that were on their bed at home
- Introduce yourself to the staff that will be working with your loved one; let them know that you are available and involved.
- Participate in care-planning meetings.
- Ensure that the nursing home is incorporating your loved one's wishes and needs into their daily care plan.

If the depression does not lessen, or gets worse, request a psychiatric evaluation from the nursing home's consultant psychiatrist or psychiatric nurse practitioner.

The home sent my dad to the ER because he struck an aide; what do I do?

When a person with dementia living in a nursing home strikes another resident or a member of the staff, a common response is for them to be sent to the nearest emergency room for an evaluation. Often there will be a request from the nursing home that the person be "psychiatrically cleared" before they return.

As we've seen throughout this chapter, the approach to take is a bit like being a detective, where you try to figure out:

- What happened? What set them off? (the triggering event)
- What can be done to decrease or eliminate the trigger?

This can be trickier when the person is living in a nursing home, especially if it's been a recent move. Since regular routine can be comforting to a person with dementia, the unfamiliar surroundings, staff they don't recognize, changing schedule, etc., provide tremendous opportunity for frustration and catastrophic responses.

When we get to Chapter 15, "Nursing Homes and Extended-Care Facilities," you'll see that even though your loved one no longer lives at home, you still need to maintain a strong presence as a caregiver—your input can make all the difference to their success at the home, since you know their needs best. You'll want to speak with the nursing home staff involved in the incident to get an idea of what actually happened. Did he get upset all at once, or has this been going on for a while?

In an ER situation, you want to make certain that, if there is something serious going on medically, it is discovered. Do not assume that much laboratory work will be obtained in the ER; often it is not. If you think your mother might have an infection, such as a urinary tract infection or pneumonia, voice your concerns and make sure they are heard. If you think the recent addition of a medication somehow altered your dad's behavior, say so.

In most instances, if nothing serious is discovered, either medically or psychiatrically, your loved one will be returned to the nursing home. There are laws that prevent nursing homes from refusing to take back a resident. However, if episodes of aggression persist—especially toward other clients—the nursing home may seek an alternative placement. If the person is admitted to the hospital, it will be important to know the rules around whether or not the nursing home must hold the person's bed and for how long.

What is normal sexual behavior in a person with dementia?

- *"My wife has Alzheimer's and still wants to have sex. I'd like to, but I don't know if it's okay?"*
- *"I moved my dad into our downstairs bedroom and on a couple occasions I've entered his room when he was masturbating. What should I do?"*
- *"Mr. Milton asked his son to bring him pornographic magazines; I don't know if we should allow him to have them in the nursing home."*

It's something of an American myth that people stop having sex—including masturbation—at some particular age. More than that, there's some stigma attached to older people and sex. However, it's well-documented that for many people, sexual activity continues into their seventies, eighties, and nineties. The preferred type of sexual activity may change for a variety of reasons, such as loss of a partner, lack of privacy, or preference, but sexual activity can and does persist.

Some people with dementing illnesses will stop engaging in sexual activities as their illness progresses; it is as though they have lost interest or have forgotten about sex. For others, they will continue to seek out physical intimacy or engage in solitary sexual activity—this is normal. What becomes a challenge are the new circumstances—living situations, physical limitations, lack of a willing partner, limited privacy, etc.—that the person with dementia now faces.

The answers as to what constitutes normal that you arrive at will be based on your personal beliefs, preferences, and the realities of your situation. What follows are some basic guidelines that should help.

- It must be consensual. Both partners must want to engage in sex. There should be no force or coercion. If you and your partner both still desire and find pleasure in physical intimacy—even though one of you has dementia—this is okay.
- There needs to be adequate privacy.
- In institutional settings, such as nursing homes and rest homes, it's important to understand their rules and how they need to balance the individual's need for some form of sexual activity with protecting other residents from unwanted advances or exposure.

Why has my father started exposing himself to others?

Sexually inappropriate behavior can occur in between 7–25 percent of individuals with dementia. It is more frequent in men and can take a number of forms, including:

- Sexually vulgar and suggestive language and propositioning others for sexual favors
- Sexual acts that can include masturbating in front of others, or masturbating excessively—to the point of injury. It might also include unwanted touching or grabbing.
- Other behaviors, such as watching pornography when others are around and don't want—or should not be allowed, as in the case of minors—to see it.

Why these behaviors occur is not completely understood, but you can try to figure out what might be triggering them. First, try to determine if the behavior is truly abnormal, or if it has more to do with the person's life situation changing. A move from their own home to a relative's house or institution, a loss of a partner, or a loss of privacy may now limit their ability to engage in various normal sexual activities. Because of this, what had been in the range of normal might now be considered a problem or inappropriate, based on the caregiver's beliefs and the physical realities of the new environment.

Next, consider any medical conditions that might account for these new behaviors. High on the list are strokes in various regions of the brain that can lead to impulsive and sexual behavior. If the person has a prior history of bipolar disorder, increased sexual behavior is often associated with the manic or "high" phases of the illness.

Or could there be cues in the environment that are being misinterpreted by a person with dementia? *"Come on Mr. Jones, it's time to go take our bath."* Maybe the aide or nurse is using terms such as, *"honey"* or *"sweetie,"* or referring to the patient as *"My boy friend."* To a person with dementia, having an attractive caregiver help you undress, use terms of endearment, and begin to touch you could be interpreted as sexual overtures. After all, earlier in their life these kinds of things were likely associated with foreplay.

How do I handle sexually inappropriate behavior?

Once it's been determined that the behavior is in fact inappropriate—at least to the situation or setting—you need to try and find ways to decrease or eliminate it. As with other problem behaviors, it's helpful to try and figure out why they're happening and start to look for ways to decrease or eliminate that trigger.

- Could the sexual behavior be related to a new medical problem or medication?
  - Certain medications, such as the benzodiazepines (valium-type drugs) can have a disinhibiting affect. If you've noticed a cause-and-effect relationship between a change in medication and a new or worsened behavior, bring this to the attention of your practitioner and consider either decreasing or changing the medication.
  - A new behavior may also indicate an acute medical problem such as a delirium (see Chapter 3). Finding and treating the cause of this may get the behavior to stop.
- If someone with dementia is trying to get in bed with someone else, it might be less about sex and more about the fact that they shared a bed for their entire adult life.
  - If this is happening in a convalescent home, it might be important to move the person to a private room, possibly one that is closer to the nursing station. This way, if they wander out in the night they can more easily be directed back to their own room.

- ◆ In a private home, strategies might include having other family members lock their bedroom doors at night or giving the person with dementia a large stuffed toy to sleep with.
- If the person is becoming aroused and trying to grab or fondle their caregiver during showering, toileting, or dressing, it may be because these activities—when done with another person in the past—have been sexual. Finding ways to diminish the sexual cues could help decrease or eliminate the behavior. One solution would be to have the caregiver for these activities be of the gender that the person is not typically attracted to. It's also important that caregivers be aware of how they're using their voice and physical touch, as they may inadvertently be sending sexual cues that are being misinterpreted.
- If the person, as a result of stroke or other brain injury, uses profane language, exposes themselves, disrobes, or masturbates in public places or excessively, it will be necessary to gently and firmly tell them to stop the behavior and redirect them to another activity. Using rewards for more positive behavior, and doing so in a consistent manner, may decrease the unwanted behavior.
- Finally, if behavioral interventions do not work, or work well enough, you may want to consider asking your medical practitioner to consider medications that might help. While there are few studies looking at this, a number of medications may decrease a person's sex drive (libido), or actually target and decrease sex hormones. In addition to the cholinesterase inhibitors and memantine (discussed in Chapter 8), some medications that have been tried for this (all off label uses) include antidepressants, antipsychotics, and hormones that diminish testosterone levels.

Chapter 10

KEEPING YOUR LOVED ONE SAFE

- How do you balance keeping someone safe with their need for independence?
- How do I get my mother to take her medications on time and correctly?
- What can I do to decrease the risk of falls?
- How can I be sure that my father is taking care of his bills?
- How can I prevent my mother from becoming a victim of identity theft?
- How do I know when I have to stop driving?
- What can I do if my father insists on driving?
- What can I do if my mother refuses to let my father stop driving?
- How can I encourage my father to leave the house now that he's lost his license?
- How do I handle my father wandering out of the home?
- How can I prevent my mother from starting a fire in the kitchen?
- What do I do about the burn marks on the furniture from Dad's cigarettes?
- Is it okay for my wife to drink alcohol?
- My mom has dementia and alcoholism—how do I handle this?
- What should I do to make the bathroom safe?
- Is it okay to have firearms in the home of a person with dementia?
- My dad refuses to let me get his guns out of the house; what do I do?
- What can I do to keep Mom safe if she has to go to the hospital?
- How do I know when I need around-the-clock in-home care?

How do you balance keeping someone safe with their need for independence?

This is one of the most important and basic questions of dementia, and the answers vary based on the degree of illness, the specifics of the current living situation, resources—both financial and human—and the specific safety concerns. As we go through this chapter looking at risk and safety issues, you'll need to recognize that with progressive dementias, what works this month will need to be reevaluated periodically, and that this is true regardless of whether your loved one is in your home or an institution.

Independence and the ability to do for ourselves are highly valued principles in our society. Americans are noted for prizing self-sufficiency and the ability to move around at will. These are some of our core values. As they are less able to do for themselves and others step in to help, people with dementia may view this "help" as unwanted, frustrating, and unwelcome. They may not be aware that there are things they can no longer do.

As the caregiver, you are faced with trying to maintain safety while not making the person feel as though you are treating them like a child. You may also be dealing with complex emotions around what is likely a radical change in your role—a daughter caring for a father, a husband caring for a wife, etc. (Family issues are discussed further in Chapter 18.)

An approach that can help with this ever-changing balance between safety and independence involves assessing the likelihood of danger. Constantly ask yourself what the chances are that your loved one, or someone else, will get hurt as a result of their actions.

- If there is even a low risk of severe harm with a particular activity or behavior, you will need to act. This can include:
  - Driving
  - Potential fire hazards in the kitchen

- ◆ Smoking in bed
- ◆ Taking medications inaccurately
- ◆ Access to firearms
- ◆ Wandering in unsafe situations
- ◆ Letting unsafe individuals into the home
- If the risk of harm is low and the degree of harm is minor, you may be able to let things ride for the time being.
  - ◆ Odd choices of clothing
  - ◆ Adequate, yet erratic, meal preparation
  - ◆ Messiness in the home

How do I get my mother to take her medications on time and correctly?

The saying that "every medication is a potential poison" is increasingly true when people are on multiple medications, as is often the case in older individuals. The risk of taking too much medication or forgetting to take life-sustaining medications is also high in people with dementia.

Depending on the degree of dementia, different strategies can help your loved one take their medications accurately. The following list goes from less intrusive strategies to ones that require higher levels of supervision.

- Set up a weekly pill box. These are available at most pharmacies. Select one that has large compartments, with the days of the week and the time of day clearly visible. To further decrease the risk of mixing up the days, many of these have daily compartments that can be taken out individually.
- Keep the pill box in the same place and try to tie the taking of medications in with other routine activities, such as brushing teeth in the morning and at bedtime, or taking morning medications with breakfast (of course this will need

to take into account any pills that need to be taken on an empty stomach).

- Remove old pill bottles from the home, and keep current pill bottles in a safe and secure location.
- Use a timer that will go off when medications need to be taken. Be aware that in people with dementia they may not be able to learn this new routine, so keep it as simple as possible, and test it out.
- Reminder phone calls—if pills are to be taken twice a day, you will call twice a day. *"Hi Mom, how are you doing? It's time to take your afternoon medication."*
- Consider in-home nursing visits for medication administration.
- Monitor the taking of medications yourself, and arrange a backup if you are not available.
- Hire an aide and instruct them to monitor the medication.

What can I do to decrease the risk of falls?

The greatest risk of falls is in the bathroom, where slippery and wet surfaces create hazards. Where people with dementia often have problems with gait and walking, any change in surface also creates an opportunity to trip. Impaired vision and problems with depth perception add to the risk. This is an area where an occupational therapist (OT) or physical therapist (PT) could be invaluable in coming up with practical safety solutions for you and your loved one with an in-home safety assessment.

There's quite a lot that you can do to decrease the risk of falls. The strategies you select will need to take into account the current home environment, the severity of the dementia, and the person's overall level of mobility.

Interventions might include:

- Proper shoes that fit well

- Eyeglasses of the right prescription
- Good lighting, especially at night
- Remove area rugs and keep walking passages free and clear.
- Chairs of the proper height and with sturdy arms that people can grab on to help raise themselves up. Consider purchasing a riser chair, an electric chair that helps a person safely stand. This can be especially helpful for people with arthritis and painful joints.
- A bathroom that is as close to the bedroom as possible. If not possible and the person has limited mobility, consider a bedside commode. Make sure they are able to get on and off of it without difficulty, and that it is sturdy.
- Install secure grab railings or bars in the shower and next to the toilet. Consider installing grab bars in hallways.
- Make sure that the toilet seat is at a height where the person can get on and off without difficulty.
- If the person uses a walker, make sure that they have enough room in all areas of the home where they will need to go.
    - Can they safely maneuver their walker in the bathroom?
    - Is there enough space for the walker next to the bed?
    - Can they successfully maneuver in the kitchen?
- Have a seat installed in the shower, so that the person can clean themselves while sitting down.
- Install a medical alert system in the home—such as Lifeline— where your loved one wears a button that can be used to call for help.

How can I be sure that my father is taking care of his bills?

It is common for a person to lose the ability to accurately manage their finances in the early stages of dementia. Oftentimes they will conceal this and it's something of a shock when family members learn important bills have gone unpaid and the checkbook is filled with mistakes. While we will discuss legal issues, such as power of attorney and conservatorships, in Chapter 14, you will have to help your loved one get a handle on the day-to-day finances and figure out what needs to be done. Neglect of a person's finances has broad-reaching and serious implications, from destruction of credit to problems with the Internal Revenue Service (IRS) if taxes have gone unpaid.

Again, you will need to balance the person's need for autonomy with preventing them from having their power turned off or the bank foreclosing on their home because they haven't paid the mortgage. A calm, gentle, and matter-of-fact approach is required, even if you are freaking out at the magnitude of the problem.

This may be one of the times when tempers flare, and caregivers and other family members may find themselves with strong negative emotions directed at the person with dementia. *"How could he do this to us?"* It will be important to remember that the person with dementia did not do this on purpose. Their inability to handle the finances is a sign of their disease and their brain is no longer able to handle this complex task.

As you work through unpaid or mismanaged finances, it will be important to put plans in place so that the monthly bills are taken care of as soon as they arrive. If you have not yet put formal plans in place—such as a power of attorney, conservatorship, or guardianship—it would be prudent to meet with an elder-law specialist to evaluate your options. Your loved one is no longer able to accurately handle their finances, so you or their caregiver will need to put an alternative plan in place.

How can I prevent my mother from becoming a victim of identity theft?

Older people are often the targets of fraud, and increasingly of identity theft. When someone with dementia becomes the target of a scam, the risk that they will divulge personal information such as a social security number or let a kind-sounding stranger into their home is great.

A number of things can help decrease this risk:

- See that all personal documents are shredded—versus thrown in the garbage—using a cross-cut shredder. This will include any mail that has the person's name and address on it.
- Never throw away unused checks, even if they are from accounts that were long-ago closed—shred them or in some other way ensure that they are completely destroyed.
- Thoroughly destroy any charge cards that are not used, and close down old accounts.
- Consider placing a "credit freeze" on all new accounts. This is a process available in most states where a person can inform the three credit agencies that no new accounts are to be opened for this individual without the freeze being lifted—typically done through a phone call. In some states this is free—especially if the person has already been a victim of identity fraud—or there may be a small charge.
- Monitor the monthly credit card statements and bank statements for any charges or payments that don't make sense.
- Obtain a copy of the person's credit report, and review it for any questionable transactions.

How do I know when I have to stop driving?

Most experts agree that even with early dementia, it is increasingly unsafe for the individual to drive. Studies looking at the rate of accidents and fatalities in people with even mild cognitive damage support this decision. Common driving errors made by people with dementia that can result in accidents include:

- Failure to check blind spots

- Lapses in attention and concentration
- Failure to look for oncoming traffic when making turns
- Confusion between the gas pedal and the brake
- Delayed response time
- Failing vision
- Problems with depth perception
- Problems with hand-eye coordination
- Diminished mobility of the head and neck; can't easily look to see what's coming

If your loved one has dementia—even mild dementia—getting behind the wheel of a car is not safe. While other authors discuss strategies in the very earliest stages of a dementia to let the person keep driving, typically with someone else supervising and just around the neighborhood, this is not recommended on account of the real and serious danger posed both for anyone in that car and for other drivers, pedestrians, etc. Beyond the safety concern is a pragmatic legal issue: If a person with dementia did get into an accident, and it was discovered that the family was aware of this, there could be legal ramifications in the form of lawsuits. It's best for the family to find other ways for the person with dementia to get around.

What can I do if my father insists on driving?

Many people with dementia will stop driving on their own because they feel it has become too scary or complicated. For others, giving up the car, or being told they cannot drive, can trigger all kinds of intense emotions—anger, rage, depression. Driving is a symbol of personal freedom and the loss of this privilege can feel devastating. *"How will I get around? How will I get to the doctor, or do my shopping?"*

When the person with dementia refuses to stop driving, it's a serious safety risk that needs to be addressed. There are several ways to do this, but regardless of the strategy, it's probably not going to be easy.

One approach will be to go directly to your state's Motor Vehicle Department and find out what the rules are around having driving licenses revoked—these differ from state to state. Some states have measurably decreased the rate of fatalities among older drivers through the simple practice of having in-person (versus through the mail) license renewal. This is often coupled with vision tests and shorter periods between renewals.

In other states, physicians may be required to report drivers they believe are unfit to the Department of Motor Vehicles; California and Pennsylvania have the most rigorous reporting laws. In most other states they may be encouraged, but not required, to do so. A call to your doctor can get this process started. *"Dad still refuses to give up the car. If I call the DMV he'll be furious with me; could you please do it?"*

Once the Department of Motor Vehicles has been notified, they may revoke or suspend the license until a test is completed to have it reinstated—such as a driving assessment, possibly using a driving simulator, or a thorough medical evaluation that results in a physician-signed statement saying that the person is at no increased risk. Doing all of the above can help get your loved one off the road, and it has the advantage of shifting some of the emotional burden off of you. *"Dr. Jones says you're no longer able to drive." "They're not renewing your license."* However, even after someone has had their license revoked, they may still try to get behind the wheel. Different strategies that can help include:

- Keep car keys secure and out of the hands of the person with dementia.
- Never leave a person with dementia in a car unattended.
- When they insist on driving, use distraction to try and shift them off the topic.
- Disable the vehicle when not in use. *"It must be broken...we'll have to get it fixed."*

What can I do if my mother refuses to let my father stop driving?

In some married couples, only one spouse drives. When that husband or wife develops dementia, the need for them to stop driving can have a devastating impact on the couple. Suddenly, what had been simple, everyday tasks—picking up groceries, visiting friends and relatives, going for medical appointments, etc.—are no longer possible. What commonly happens is that the well, non-driving spouse will attempt to cover for their partner and downplay the severity of their dementia. *"He's never had an accident in his life." "I'm with him all the time in case he forgets."*

Regardless, the risk of accidents, including fatal accidents, is increased, and the driver needs to be off the road. Strategies to accomplish this may include:

- A frank discussion with both your parents. Acknowledge the real loss that this represents, and also your concern that they may cause an accident, become injured, or injure someone else.
- Enlist the aid of the family physician. If necessary, ask if they could handle reporting the dementia to the Department of Motor Vehicles (DMV).
- Report directly to the DMV yourself.
- Talk with the well spouse about whether or not they would consider learning to drive. Or if they already have their license, but have stopped driving on their own, see if they would be interested in taking a driving course to brush up their skills and their confidence behind the wheel. Would they feel more comfortable if you went out with them a few times?
- Identify alternative sources of transportation that may be available, such as senior shuttles, local taxi services, and public transportation.
- Hire a driver, or find an aide service that offers transportation.

How can I encourage my father to leave the house now that he's lost his license?

In the preceding questions we looked at the dangers of a person with dementia continuing to drive and the need for them to stop. On the other side of the decision to stop driving is the difficult reality of figuring out transportation. Options for older individuals, especially those who are frail and/or disabled, are limited. Additionally, there is a strong emotional component to being dependant on others for transportation. *"I hate having to ask for favors all the time." "I feel like such a burden now that I can't get around on my own."* For people on a fixed income, taking a taxi or even public transportation may seem too expensive.

Solutions to the transportation problem will be highly individualized and based on what's available in the community, what resources the family can come up with, and the individual's ability to pay out-of-pocket. Some options might include:

- In the case of couples where only one spouse drove—and is no longer able to do so—is it possible that the other spouse could learn to drive?
- Can family or friends provide a regular weekly shopping trip? If this can be at a set time and set day every week, it decreases the anxiety and distress caused by feeling like they always have to ask for favors.
- When planning a family event, make sure that the driving arrangements for the person with dementia, or the couple that has no driver, are explicit and not left till the last minute.
- Check with you local senior centers or Council on Aging for low-cost transportation options in your community, such as "senior shuttles." These might include free transportation to and from doctor's appointments, as well as scheduled shopping trips. Keep the phone numbers and instructions clearly visible in your loved one's home.

- See what public transportation options are available in your community. For the person with dementia, you will need to assess whether or not they would be able to successfully use public transportation. This suggestion is more geared toward the well spouse.

How do I handle my father wandering out of the home?

As dementia worsens, wandering away from the home is a common problem. Often what happens is the person goes for a walk, is unable to remember how to get back home, and a dangerous and even life-threatening situation develops. Depending on the time of year, they may be walking for miles in 100-degree weather or in the middle of a blizzard, wearing nothing but a housedress. They may be lost in a dangerous neighborhood or be at risk for being struck by a car or truck as they wander down the side of the interstate in the middle of the night. Depending on the living situation and stage of dementia, there are many different approaches to address wandering. Here are a few:

- Ensure that your loved one wears an identification bracelet with their name, address, and telephone number. For $45 these are available from the Alzheimer's Association (www.alz.org). They also have a "Safe Return" program, which includes twenty-four-hour telephone assistance, should your loved one become lost.
- Let your neighbors and local police know about the risk of wandering.
- Alarm the doors in the house, so that when they are opened or closed, a bell or buzzer goes off.

How can I prevent my mother from starting a fire in the kitchen?

Like the bathroom, the kitchen will need to be modified for the person with dementia. The risk of fires from pots unattended or ovens left on is very real and needs to be addressed early on in the disease.

In early dementia, some find that switching all cooking and heating over to a microwave is helpful. This does not eliminate the risk of fire, but it does decrease it. The downside here is that if the person has not been using a microwave all along, learning the buttons may prove to be frustrating. For simple cooking and heating tasks, putting pictures over the buttons, or purchasing a microwave that already has these, may simplify the task of heating a cup of tea, baking a potato, or warming a prepared meal. Gas stoves and ovens should be safely disconnected; the risk that someone will turn on the gas and then forget to light it is too great.

Previously prepared meals that can be heated in a microwave, raw foods, and delivered meals are some options. There may be agencies in your community such as "Meals on Wheels" or "Friendly Visitors" that are able to deliver low-cost and nutritious meals.

What do I do about the burn marks on the furniture from Dad's cigarettes?

In addition to the known health hazards of cigarette smoking (cancer, lung disease, etc.), the risk for starting a fire becomes severe if someone with dementia continues to smoke. It's easy for them to forget a lit cigarette and for it to smolder and ignite a couch, bed, waste basket, or carpet.

Clearly the best solution—from both a safety and health standpoint—is to have the person stop smoking entirely. Under the direction of your medical provider, the distress from nicotine withdrawal may be diminished by using a nicotine patch (it may be too difficult to follow the instructions for nicotine gum) or other medications such as buproprion (Zyban) or varenicline (Chantix) that can help with smoking cessation.

If the person with dementia is allowed to continue smoking, it needs to be monitored. Cigarettes, matches, and lighters have to be kept safe and out of the person's possession. You might decide to create a designated smoking area in the home—a porch, deck, or yard would be ideal. This is often the approach taken in rest homes, nursing homes, and retirement homes that allow cigarette smoking.

Is it okay for my wife to drink alcohol?

Alcohol and dementia are not a good mix for several reasons:

- People become more unsteady on their feet and are at a greater risk for falls when they've been drinking.
- People with dementia will have even more difficulty performing functions and remembering things if they've been drinking.
- Alcohol is disinhibiting and can lead to unwanted behaviors—wandering, irritability, aggressiveness, and sexual behaviors.
- Alcohol can interact with many medications the person is taking. This is especially true for any sedating or tranquilizing medications. The combination with alcohol could lead to excess sedation, unsteadiness, and, in extreme circumstances, even decrease the person's ability to breathe.

All of that said, for someone with an early dementia who is not on medication that would interact with alcohol, an occasional glass of wine or beer with friends or family is probably okay. However, if the person seems unsteady on their feet or their behavior is adversely affected by the drink, it's best to eliminate it entirely.

One halfway measure some caregivers have found is the use of non-alcoholic wine and beer. While some of these still contain a tiny amount of alcohol, they should be safe in moderation.

My mom has dementia and alcoholism—how do I handle this?

- *"It wasn't until my dad went into the hospital that I found all of the booze bottles. He'd hidden them all around the house. Growing up we knew he drank, but he always kept it from us, and he never seemed that drunk. I've now come to find out he's been walking to the store every morning and getting a fifth of bourbon."*

- *"My wife and I have always had a couple of Manhattans in the evening. Her favorite expression used to be, 'it's always five o'clock somewhere.' I guess maybe she wouldn't always stop at two. Now I think she's sneaking drinks in the morning to keep her hands from shaking."*

Alcoholism can affect people of all ages. It's fairly common in the course of evaluating someone for dementia to find that the person has a problem with alcohol, and has been a daily or heavy drinker and may be alcohol-dependent. In instances of people who have been drinking heavily for many years, alcohol can actually lead to a form of dementia (see Chapter 5).

When someone is physically dependant on alcohol—usually a daily and/or heavy drinker—their body can go through a dangerous withdrawal syndrome if they should just stop drinking cold turkey. Alcohol withdrawal typically starts a day to two days after the last drink, but in some instances of heavy drinkers—especially those who have been drinking throughout the day—a withdrawal can start hours after the last drink. For some the withdrawal may be delayed and not occur until three or even four days after the last drink.

In mild cases, withdrawal presents with symptoms of nervousness, anxiety, and depression. But alcohol withdrawal can be severe and even deadly, with a condition known as delirium tremens or the DTs. When someone withdraws from alcohol, their blood pressure and pulse can shoot up. They may become shaky and tremulous and are at risk for having seizures. Hallucinations are a symptom of serious withdrawal, as are severe confusion and disorientation. Auditory and tactile hallucinations—hearing things that aren't there and feeling things crawling on your skin—can also be a part of the withdrawal syndrome.

The disease of alcoholism needs to be taken seriously and treated safely. If you suspect that someone you are caring for is alcohol-dependent, they will need to be evaluated for a medically managed detoxification. Depending on the severity of the person's alcoholism and what other medical conditions they might have, the detoxification may need to happen in a hospital.

Once the detoxification is complete—a few days to a couple of weeks—the person should be safe from symptoms of withdrawal. Depending on their living situation, degree of dementia, etc., the challenge now is to keep them from returning to the bottle. If there is alcohol in the home, it needs to be locked away. Mouthwashes and other over-the-counter medications that contain alcohol—and many do—need to be removed. In general, you'll need to think through any possible access to alcohol and try to eliminate it. If the person has been walking to the liquor store, have a word with the store owner. If the person with dementia has had a friend, family member, or neighbor bring them alcohol, you'll need to let that person know that it needs to stop. If the person has been drinking in a bar or with friends at the golf club, you'll need to find ways to prevent that from happening.

Should the person again start drinking, it will be important to have them medically evaluated, especially if there is a history of alcohol withdrawal. As a result of the dementia and the memory loss, it's unlikely they will remember they have a problem with alcohol, and so vigilance on the part of the caregiver(s) is critical.

What should I do to make the bathroom safe?

Bathroom safety needs to take into account a number of factors: the physical and mental status of the person with dementia, and the actual bathroom. General safety tips that can make a bathroom more secure, especially if someone becomes light-headed when standing or are unsteady on their feet, include:

- Grab bars in the shower and along the walls. These need to be properly installed so they can take the person's weight if need be.
- Make sure that the flooring is slip-resistant; avoid area rugs the person can trip on.
- Use non-slip adhesive on the floor of the bath and/or shower.
- Consider removing any raised flooring structures—such as saddles that connect one room's flooring to the next—if they represent a tripping hazard.
- Be sure there is adequate lighting in all areas of the bathroom, including the shower stall.
- Go through the medicine cabinet and remove all old medications and any product that could be mistaken for something edible.
- Keep the walkways clear. If there are any obstacles in front of the shower, toilet, sink, or tub, remove them. If the person uses a walker, be sure they have unobstructed pathways and adequate room to maneuver—such as turning around to get on and off the toilet.

- Ensure that the toilet seat is at the right height. For many people with arthritis or degenerative joint disease that involves the knees and hips, getting up and down can be hard. If the seat is higher, this decreases the amount of lift a person will need to generate with their arms.
- A grab bar next to the toilet or a special raised toilet seat that incorporates arm rails may help with getting up and down.
- A shower or bath seat allows the person to wash while in a seated position.
- Adjust the hot-water thermostat lower so that the person is not able to get scalded accidentally.
- Be sure there are no electrical appliances in the bathroom that could be a hazard for electrocution.
- If the person's dementia has progressed to where they are not able to perform all the steps needed in the bathroom, they will need someone to help them along and prompt them through the various processes of bathing, showering, and toileting (for particular strategies with these personal hygiene tasks, see Chapter 9).
- Consider purchasing and installing a walk-in tub.

Is it okay to have firearms in the home of a person with dementia?

Firearms in the home take on a heightened level of risk for the person with dementia harming themselves or someone else. It is a fact that the single highest-risk group for suicide in this country is older white men. By far, the most common method of suicide is with a firearm. Having a gun in the home of a person with dementia, no matter how safely kept, represents added risk.

Additional risks for committing suicide in this group include being widowed or divorced, and having recently been diagnosed with a serious illness. This profile clearly fits many with dementia, and the period of highest risk is when someone is still able to think clearly enough (early or mild dementia) to put a suicidal impulse into action.

Beyond the risk of suicide and self-harm is the added concern that the person with dementia will hurt somebody else, either accidentally or in response to misperceiving their actions. *"I heard noises downstairs...I thought someone had broken in."* If even after knowing the risk you decide to keep firearms in the house, it is vitally important that they are locked at all times in a vault or gun safe; that ammunition is not kept with the firearm; and that firearms are never left loaded. But clearly, the best strategy is to remove all firearms from the home.

My dad refuses to let me get his guns out of the house; what do I do?

"I've been a hunter my entire life. I keep my shotguns locked up. You're not taking them out of my house!"

Each state has statutes around owning firearms. Some states will have specific restrictions around people who have mental disabilities such as dementia purchasing or owning firearms. Regardless, if your loved one with dementia has firearms in the home and is unwilling to let you remove them, here are some things you can do:

- See if the person has any plans for the guns, such as giving them to a relative or selling them. Offer to do this for them:
  - *"Why not give them to John now? He'd really like that?"*
  - *"I'd be happy to handle the sale and then we can buy you something you want with the money."*
- Contact your local police or sheriff to find out what the rules are in your state about removing firearms. If you have specific concerns that your loved one is unsafe around the firearms, let them know that.

What can I do to keep Mom safe if she has to go to the hospital?

Hospitals can be dangerous places; it's estimated that between 40,000–90,000 people die annually from medical mistakes in hospitals. Beyond this, the risk for acquiring antibiotic-resistant infections is greatly increased in a hospital. When your loved one requires hospitalization, this is a time for increased vigilance. You will need to be certain that the treating physicians and nurses are aware of all medications, including dosages and frequency, your loved one is taking. As the person with dementia might not be able to provide a thorough medical history that includes past surgeries, allergies, and other active medical problems, it will be up to you to do this. You might want to consider keeping an updated copy of your loved one's medical history, or a completed questionnaire such as the one in Appendix C, that you can print out and give to the treating medical team.

Throughout the hospital stay it is important that you stay in close contact with the treatment team (doctors, nurses, social worker). As medications get added or changed, be sure that you understand why. Speak up and do not be afraid to ask questions. If you see a problem, do not assume that someone else—a doctor or nurse—has already identified it. Bring it to the attention of the staff.

- *"My dad's intravenous site seems awfully red; is that normal?"*
- *"My husband is getting a bad sore on his back; could somebody look at that?"*
- *"What's that fluid in the IV bag?"*
- *"Mom seems a lot more confused today; this isn't her normal state."*
- *"He seems to be in an awful lot of pain; do they know the cause?"*
- *"You can't just leave the meal tray in front of him, or he won't eat a thing. Someone needs to feed him and make sure he takes adequate liquids."*

It's okay, and often necessary, to be the squeaky wheel. Remember, you know this person far better than these professionals. Your input, oversight, and concern will help your loved one get the medical attention they require as safely and quickly as possible.

How do I know when I need around-the-clock in-home care?

- *"It's gotten to where the minute I leave her alone, she's out the door. Thank God we put the global-positioning device on her, but the police are getting upset with how often they have to call for someone to pick her up."*
- *"He won't eat if someone's not there. And the bathroom is a nightmare; he's been using the garbage pail as a toilet. I've had to disconnect the stove, but I worry constantly that he'll have an accident or do something to harm himself."*
- *"Her arthritis is so bad she can't even get out of bed without someone helping. If I'm not on it constantly she starts to develop horrible bed sores from lying in bed all day long."*

Around-the-clock in-home care/supervision, whether provided by family, friends, or a paid caregiver, is an option that many choose for people with moderate to severe dementia who would otherwise require placement in a nursing home. The decision to provide around-the-clock care usually centers on safety or health concerns, though of course there is a financial question as well. Some examples of conditions that make around-the-clock in-home care necessary include:

- The person is too unsteady on their feet. They need someone to assist with helping them get around the house, get in and out of bed, onto the toilet, into a chair, etc.
- The person is too medically fragile to be alone.

- The person's behavior is too unpredictable and dangerous for them to be left alone—they habitually wander out of the house, are at risk for setting fires, continually try to get behind the wheel of a car despite moderate or advanced dementia, etc.
- The person's ADLs—eating, dressing, toileting, walking, washing—have deteriorated to where they need available help throughout the day and night.

Chapter 11

UNDERSTANDING MEDICARE

- What is Medicare and who is eligible for it?
- My brother is fifty-five and has early-onset Alzheimer's; can he get covered by Medicare?
- What are the different parts of Medicare?
- Why is Medicare so confusing?
- How do I get Medicare A?
- How do I get Medicare B?
- What kinds of things aren't covered by Medicare A and B?
- How does Medicare D work?
- So what do I really save with Medicare D?
- Even with Medicare D I can't afford all of my medications—what do I do?
- How much does Medicare cover?
- What are Medicare Advantage Plans?
- What is managed Medicare?
- What is supplemental Medicare coverage (Medigap)?
- Does someone need to be homebound to receive Medicare in-home services?
- Can people with dementia and Alzheimer's get in-home services under Medicare?
- Who determines if something is medically necessary?
- What can I do if Medicare refuses to pay for services or denies a claim?

What is Medicare and who is eligible for it?

Medicare is a federally funded health care benefit for people over the age of sixty-five who have worked for more than ten years for a Medicare-covered employer; it's also for younger individuals with disabilities, such as early-onset Alzheimer's and other dementias. It is also for people of any age with severe kidney disease that requires either dialysis treatment or kidney transplant.

There are a number of excellent web sites that provide extensive information, as well as free government publications on Medicare. These include:

- Medicare itself: visit www.medicare.gov, or call 1–800–633–4227 (TTY 1–877–486–2048)
- The Social Security Administration online—you can access their one-hundred-plus-page Medicare manual, including large-print format, at http://www.ssa.gov/mediinfo.htm, or call 1–800–772–1213 (TTY 1–800–325–0778)
- The Centers for Medicare and Medicaid Services (CMS). This was previously the Healthcare Finance Administration (HCFA). http://www.cms.hhs.gov
- The Center for Medicare Advocacy, Inc.—a non-profit organization that provides education, advocacy, and legal assistance around Medicare-related issues. www.medicareadvocacy.org, or call 1–860–456–7790

My brother is fifty-five and has early-onset Alzheimer's; can he get covered by Medicare?

For people younger than sixty-five with disabilities, including early-onset Alzheimer's and other dementing illnesses, eligibility for Medicare is tied to Social Security Disability Insurance (SSDI). This means you must first be deemed eligible and receive SSDI before becoming eligible for the Medicare disability benefit. To be considered eligible for SSDI, the individual must be considered disabled for at least twelve months, or diagnosed with a disability that is expected to last at least twelve months, have worked at a job long enough and recently enough, and have paid payroll (FICA) taxes. Once considered disabled, Medicare coverage will begin after twenty-four months.

- Information on SSDI eligibility and starter kits are available through the Department of Social Services (DSS), www.socialsecurity.gov, or call 1–800–772–1213 (TTY 1–800–325–0778)
- Information on Medicare eligibility is available from the Centers for Medicare and Medicaid Services (CMS) http://www.cms.hhs.gov, or call 1–877–267–2323 (TTY 1–866–226–1819)

It is common for people applying to SSDI to be turned down on their first application. Persistence is important and additional guidance can be obtained through the Alzheimer's association (www.alz.org,) or you might consider hiring an attorney with expertise in disability law.

What are the different parts of Medicare?

In this and the following questions we'll break each of the major parts of Medicare—A, B, C, and D—down into what they cover and an approximation of how much they will pay for different services, facilities, and medical equipment.

Medicare A, often referred to as the "inpatient benefit," covers:

- Hospitalization
- A convalescent or Skilled Nursing Facility (SNF)—but not the long-term care or custodial care that is often needed with dementia. In order to use this benefit, a person must have previously been in a hospital for at least three days with a related illness. An example might be someone who has broken

a hip, had it repaired, and now needs four to six weeks in a nursing/rehabilitation facility to regain their ability to walk. Another example could be someone who has had a stroke and requires several weeks of rehabilitation and therapy to regain functioning.

- In-home nursing services (home health care). This can include nursing services, home health aides, social work services, and occupational and physical therapy.
- Hospice care—end-of-life care for those with terminal illnesses who are expected to live six months or less
- Durable medical equipment such as wheelchairs, walkers, oxygen, etc.

Medicare B handles more of the outpatient side of things, including various tests and procedures that your physician might order from her office. It also covers some in-home services not covered by Medicare A. Medicare B also helps with ambulance services and screening and preventative tests, such as bone mass measurement for osteoporosis, colorectal screenings for cancer, and prostate, diabetes, and heart disease screenings. Medicare B also covers an annual flu shot, other immunizations, yearly mammograms, and cervical cancer screenings. Medicare B will pay for a one-time physical examination if it's obtained within six months of signing up for part B. Be aware that co-pays and/or a deductible may apply for any of these services.

Medicare C, also known as "Medicare Advantage Plans," are private insurance providers that are approved by Medicare and work using health maintenance organization (HMO) or preferred-provider organization (PPO) models. Typically, this means you will need to use physicians and facilities within their provider network. If you elect to go with a part C plan, it will combine your part A and part B benefits. Your out-of-pocket expenses under a part C plan may be different than under regular Medicare. Medicare C plans must also include emergency services, even if delivered outside of their provider network.

Medicare D is the recently enacted (2006) pharmaceutical benefit that helps defray the cost of paying for medicines, especially if the individual meets criteria for being below or near the poverty level.

Why is Medicare so confusing?

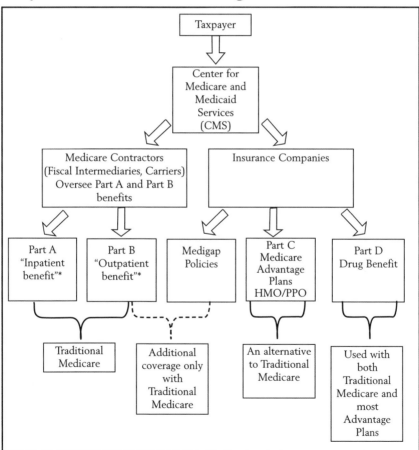

If you find yourself scratching your head while trying to figure out which Medicare coverage is best for you and/or your loved one, you're not alone. Medicare, which was signed into law in 1965 largely to ensure that older Americans have health care coverage, has undergone numerous revisions over the years. The more recent changes that have led to the creation of Medicare Part C (Medicare Advantage Plans) and Medicare Part D (prescription drug benefit) have moved the Medicare system more into the private sector—that is, less direct government control and various insurance companies offering a vast array of products. In addition, there has been a general trend to shift more of the cost for Medicare onto the beneficiary through higher co-pays, deductibles, and premiums. There is considerable debate as to whether recent changes have improved matters, or just made them more confusing and expensive for both the Medicare beneficiary and the taxpayer.

Before the addition of Parts C and D, deciding on Medicare coverage used to be a relatively straightforward process where most people would automatically get Medicare A (the inpatient benefit) and enroll for Medicare B (professional services, outpatient visits, etc.) This is called "traditional Medicare," and if they could afford it people would purchase gap coverage (Medigap) to defray the cost of co-payments and deductibles.

Now people are faced with many more options that can render the entire process stressful and confusing. People now must decide if they should opt for traditional Medicare, or if there is a Medicare Advantage plan (Part C) that makes more sense. They must also sort through the Medicare Part D plan and decide which they should pick, or if they already have drug coverage, if it's better to stay with that. In many states there can be more than a dozen Medicare D plans offered, and all of them might be quite different.

While it's not possible to make a black-or-white recommendation, in general most people will get the broadest coverage through sticking with traditional Medicare, where they can see any provider and use any facility that accepts Medicare payment. For many, augmenting this with gap coverage (Medigap) will also make sense.

How do I get Medicare A?

Most people automatically get Medicare Part A coverage for free when they turn sixty-five because they or their spouse paid Medicare taxes when they were working. If you are not eligible for free Medicare Part A you may be able to buy it, but this will typically involve purchasing Medicare Part B, as well.

As the "normal retirement" age (the age at which you are eligible for full benefits) for social security increases to sixty-seven—for those born after 1960—more people will need to enroll for Medicare A instead of having it begin automatically with the start of their social security. If you were born before 1937 you are still automatically enrolled at age sixty-five, but for everyone in between it has also gone to age sixty-seven. To enroll for Medicare A, you will need to call Social Security at 1–800–772–1213 and speak with a representative about enrolling in Medicare, but not Social Security. They will assist with the application and will require you to submit proof of age, typically your birth certificate.

A chart of "normal retirement" age based on year of birth is available at the social security website: www.socialsecurity.gov/retire2/retirechart.htm.

How do I get Medicare B?

Unlike Medicare A, which most people will get for free at age sixty-five, you need to enroll for Medicare B. In many ways, Medicare B is more like a typical insurance plan, in which you will have an annual deductible and monthly premiums. People who plan to sign up for Medicare B are encouraged to do so when they first become eligible, usually at age sixty-five. If people don't sign up but want to do so later, there is a 10 percent penalty added to their premiums for every year they could have enrolled but didn't.

A recent change to Medicare B is that the monthly premiums will now be based (as of January 2007) on your income. This mostly affects individuals who earn at least $80,000 and couples with joint incomes greater than $160,000. For more information about enrolling for Medicare B, call 1–800–633–4227 (TTY 1–877–486–2048).

What kinds of things aren't covered by Medicare A and B?

For medical services and equipment to be covered under Medicare A and/or B, they need to be deemed "medically necessary" by a physician (generally a Doctor of Medicine—MD—or Doctor of Osteopathy—DO) or other approved licensed independent practitioner (LIP). Even with this designation, however, many important medical procedures and examinations are not covered under Medicare A or B. For those people who opt out of A and B and instead go with a commercial Medicare C plan, it is often these uncovered services—such as being able to get eye care and glasses or a hearing aid—that steers their decision. The following list, while not exhaustive, contains some of the items not usually covered by Medicare A and B:

- Dental services, including dentures
- Medications (these may be covered under Medicare part D)
- Cosmetic procedures (plastic surgery)
- Hearing aids, hearing examinations, and hearing tests
- Eye examinations and glasses (may be covered for some conditions)
- Foot care (trimming of calluses and corns)
- Routine physical examinations (this does not refer to the one-time "Welcome to Medicare" examination)

- Long-term residential or custodial care as is often needed with Alzheimer's and dementia
- Acupuncture
- Chiropractic services (there are some exceptions)

How does Medicare D work?

Medicare D—prescription drug coverage—is the most recent addition to Medicare. You also need to be aware that even with Medicare D the out-of-pocket expense for medications, for most people, will still be considerable. Understanding Medicare D can be confusing and deciding what makes the most sense for you will be based on a number of factors.

If you have traditional Medicare (Parts A and B) you can sign up for a part D prescription drug plan through different insurance companies that offer them. These vary from state to state. Most plans—although not all—will have a deductible and charge a monthly premium. Even after you have paid the deductibles, most of these plans will only cover a percentage of the cost.

If you have Medicare C/Medicare Advantage Plan (instead of A and B), your particular HMO or PPO may offer prescription drug coverage as part of your overall plan, or as an add-on for which you will pay an additional monthly premium.

To assist in choosing a Medicare D plan, you can see your options online at www.medicare.gov; go to "Compare Medicare Prescription Drug Plans." You can also call 1–800–633–4222 (TTY 1–877–486–2048). There are a number of important factors that will guide you in your decision, including:

- Are the drugs you need covered under a particular plan?
- Can you use your pharmacy? Not all plans allow you to use every pharmacy.
- If you already have prescription drug coverage through

another insurer (employer or union), be very careful—signing up for Medicare D could nullify this benefit.

- What are the actual out-of-pocket expenses for you? Be sure to consider monthly premiums, deductibles, the percentage you will be expected to pay for medications, and the cost of generic versus name-brand medications.

So what do I really save with Medicare D?

Let's break down the out-of-pocket yearly cost for someone who has a Medicare D prescription plan and traditional Medicare (parts A and B). The dollar amounts may vary slightly based on the prescription plan you choose. Amounts used in the following are taken from *Medicare and You 2007*, a free publication from the Centers for Medicare and Medicaid Services.

1. Yearly deductible: $265. This is the first amount spent on medications, and you pay it in full.
2. After the deductible the plan will pick up a percentage of prescription drug costs, until you reach a limit of $2,400. The percentage you pay versus what they pay will be based on the plan you have selected. A typical plan will cover 80 percent, with you picking up the other 20 percent.
3. After the $2,400 limit has been reached, you have entered a "coverage gap"—also known as the donut hole—where you will now need to pay the full cost of prescription medications until you reach a second ceiling. Your out-of-pocket expense for the donut hole is $3,051.25.
4. After you have reached this ceiling and paid a total of $3,850 out of pocket (this includes your deductible, monthly premiums, coverage gap, etc.), you have entered "catastrophic coverage" where you will be expected to pay either a minimal

percentage (5 percent) or small co-pay per prescription.

5. You also need to be aware that there is an enrollment penalty if you do not sign up for Medicare D within your initial enrollment period. This penalty will continue as long as you have Medicare D. The penalty is calculated by taking 1 percent of the national average premium and then multiplying it by the number of months you were eligible but did not enroll.

Even with Medicare D I can't afford all of my medications—what do I do?

For people who fall near or below the poverty level, there is special assistance available for prescription drugs. Similarly, if you have already been receiving medication coverage through your state's Medicaid program, you will automatically be enrolled in a Part D plan with little or no out-of-pocket expense for prescription drugs.

To find out if you or the person you are caring for qualify for special assistance, you can apply online at www.socialsecurity.gov and follow the link for "Medicare Prescription Drug Plan." You could also call the Social Security Administration at 1–800–772–1213 (TTY 1–800–325–0778).

Many states also offer assistance with medication for people who do not meet the poverty levels needed to be eligible for Medicaid. To find out more contact your area Agency on Aging.

How much does Medicare cover?

Your actual out-of-pocket cost for various medical services, procedures, and equipment will vary based on whether or you have just Medicare A, Medicare A and B, or have opted for a Medicare Advantage Plan (Medicare C). If you have questions about what you will be expected to pay for a hospital stay, trip to the doctor, lab work, etc., it's a good idea to speak with the hospital's billing department or someone in your physician's office who can answer your specific questions. It's also important to know that hospitals and medical providers who accept Medicare as payment can only charge up to a rate that is set by the Center for Medicare and Medicaid Services (CMS)—this is referred to as the "Medicare Approved Rate."

Taking figures provided in the official 2007 CMS publication, *Medicare and You*, we get some guidelines about your out-of-pocket expense. Remember that, in order for any service to be covered by Medicare, it must be deemed "medically necessary."

Medicare A costs are:
Medicare B costs are:

Blood	You pay for the first three pints of blood as an inpatient and then 20% of the Medicare approved amount for additional blood (unless you've donated your own, in anticipation of a surgery or other procedure—called an autologous donation).
Home Health Care	You pay nothing for medically necessary services.
	You pay 20% of the Medicare approved amount for covered durable medical equipment.
Hospice Care	You pay up to a $5 co-pay for prescriptions.
	You pay 5% of the Medicare-approved amount for inpatient respite care.
Hospital Stays	You pay a $992 deductible and no co-pay for the first 60 days in each benefit period.
	After the first 60 days you pay $248 per day up until day 90.
	After day 90 you pay $496 per "lifetime reserve day."
Nursing Home/Skilled Nursing Facility	You pay nothing for the first 20 days in a given benefit period.
	You pay $124 per day for days 21–100.
	You cover all costs after day 100.

Annual deductible	You pay the first $131 annually.
Blood	You pay for the first three pints of blood as an outpatient and then 20% of the Medicare approved amount for additional (unless you've donated your own—autologous donation).
Laboratory Services (blood draws, urine tests, etc.)	You pay nothing for approved services.
Home Health Services	You pay nothing for medically necessary services.
	You pay 20% of the Medicare approved amount for covered durable medical equipment.
Medical and other Services	You pay 20% of the Medicare approved amount for most outpatient doctor visits.
Mental Health/Behavioral Health services	You pay 50% of the Medicare approved amount.
Outpatient Hospital services	You pay a co-pay that varies by service.

What are Medicare Advantage Plans?

While not available everywhere, Medicare Advantage Plans (Part C) are an alternative to traditional Medicare. These plans take various forms, such as health maintenance organizations (HMOs), preferred provider organizations (PPOs), fee-for-service plans, and Medicare Special Needs Plans (SNPs). The decision to choose a Medicare Advantage Plan will often have to do with benefits covered by the plan that are not covered under traditional Medicare, such as eyeglasses, dental coverage, and prescription coverage. There may also be lower deductibles and/or co-pays. Depending on the plan you choose you may be restricted to seeing physicians and medical providers (preferred providers) covered by the plan.

To enroll for a Medicare Advantage Plan you will need to have both Medicare A and B. You will continue to pay your part B premium to Medicare, and you may also have to pay a premium for the C plan you have chosen. Medigap policies (see page 167) do not work with Medicare Advantage plans—they will not pick up the co-pays and deductibles. So for people who choose a Medicare Advantage Plan, there is little sense in continuing to purchase Medigap coverage.

What is managed Medicare?

Whenever the word "managed" is connected with health insurance (including Medicare and Medicaid), it means that some insurance company is providing oversight—often referred to as utilization review—for the benefit. While all Medicare plans, even original Medicare A and B plans, have oversight, the term managed Medicare mostly refers to Medicare Advantage plans (see previous question).

In a managed Medicare Plan—versus traditional Medicare—the following may apply:

- You need to use physicians, facilities, and medical providers in your plan's list. This is different from traditional Medicare, where you can see any provider that accepts Medicare reimbursement.
- Treatment and tests may need to be "preauthorized" or "approved" by the insurance company.
- It's important to know which hospital(s) are on your plan. Some plans will only cover certain hospitals, or there may be higher co-pays and deductibles should you not be admitted to their preferred institution.

- The length of a hospital stay will be closely monitored by the insurance company. Medical providers may be required to have frequent contacts with your plan's manager should you require additional time in the hospital.

What is supplemental Medicare coverage (Medigap)?

Supplemental Medicare coverage, sometimes referred to as Medigap, is insurance offered by private companies to pay for the co-pays and deductibles not covered by traditional Medicare (Parts A and B). Medigap polices vary in cost, but offer a standardized coverage. All Medigap policies will clearly state that they are "Medicare Supplement Insurance." They do not pick up the co-pays and deductibles for Medicare Advantage Plans (Part C).

To find out more about Medigap policies, you can call 1–800–633–4227 and ask for a free copy of the publication *Choosing a Medigap Policy: A Guide to Health Insurance for People with Medicare.*

Does someone need to be homebound to receive Medicare in-home services?

Yes; however, the Medicare definition of "homebound" is open to some interpretation. In general the person must be mostly confined to the home, but they are allowed to go out for necessary medical appointments, important family events, and even the occasional trip to the hairdresser.

Can people with dementia and Alzheimer's get in-home services under Medicare?

The quick answer is yes; Medicare does cover in-home services for people with chronic conditions such as a dementia. However, in order to receive in-home services there must be some element of "skilled care." Skilled care is provided by or under the supervision of particular professionals, such as registered nurses (RNs), licensed practical nurses (LPNs), and occupational, physical, and speech therapists. The skilled services provided must be medically necessary and cannot be things that could be performed by a family member, friend, or unskilled person. In addition, the in-home services must be under a frequently reviewed treatment plan (overseen by an MD or doctor of osteopathy) that has specific goals and objectives that are designed to improve function, maintain function, or slow or prevent further deterioration.

Who determines if something is medically necessary?

In the Medicare system, medical necessity is determined by the licensed professional who has ordered the service. This is most typically a physician, but could also be a nurse practitioner, licensed psychologist (PhD) and, for some services, a licensed clinical social worker (LCSW) or physician's assistant (PA). The professional who orders any medical service under Medicare—it could be a lab test, a visit from a nurse, a procedure, etc.—by signing their name to the treatment plan, lab slip, or order sheet attests to the medical necessity of what is being ordered.

What can I do if Medicare refuses to pay for services or denies a claim?

- *"Mom's visiting nurse services were denied by Medicare. They said that they weren't 'medically necessary.'"*
- *"The aide said she can't come anymore because Medicare won't pay for her."*

If you receive a claim denial from Medicare (it will in fact come from the Medicare contractor) there will be contact information on it about how to file an appeal. Most claims will be denied around issues related to the "medical necessity" of the procedure or test; having the prescribing physician document why the particular service is indeed medically necessary will help with the appeal process. This can be done by attaching a note from the physician to the appeal/redetermination paperwork—remember to keep copies of everything. There will also be a 120-day time limit for filing from the time you receive the denial.

For people with dementia, a denial may be based on not having measurable goals and objectives for a particular service—often an in-home service—that is ordered to show improvement, such as occupational therapy or physical therapy. This can be appealed; it is something of a myth that services must move toward measurable improvement. This is not the case and if a service can help maintain function, and is deemed medically necessary by the prescribing physician, it should be covered.

If the appeal is turned down there will be a process for resubmitting, and if you are again turned down and believe the service should be covered, your case can be referred for an administrative law judge hearing. And even after this, if the claim is denied, there are further avenues for pursuing the claim at increasingly higher levels, to a Determination Appeals Board or eventually a Judicial Review.

A couple of things to keep in mind: each level of appeal must be filed within a specified time frame—the clock starts ticking from the minute you receive the latest denial. Also, you may want to consider legal assistance if you believe you are being denied a service that should be covered under your Medicare benefit.

Agencies that might be able to assist include:
- The Center for Medicare Advocacy
  National Office, Connecticut
  P. O. Box 350, Willimantic, CT 06226

Tel: 860–456–7790
Website: www.medicareadvocacy.org
- Your state's legal aid office
- Your local area agency on aging

Chapter 12

UNDERSTANDING MEDICAID

- What is Medicaid?
- What does Medicaid pay for?
- How does someone become eligible for Medicaid?
- What is a Medicaid spend-down?
- Will my mom lose the house if Dad has to go onto Medicaid?
- What other assets can Dad keep if Mom is on Medicaid and in a nursing home?

What is Medicaid?

Medicaid, which is the largest payer for nursing-home-level care in the United States, is a program that provides health insurance to low-income families and others who fall below state-designated financial guidelines. This includes children of low-income families, some older Americans—especially those requiring nursing-home-level care—and people with disabilities, including psychiatric disabilities, that fall below a certain income and resource level.

Unlike Medicare, which is fully funded by the federal government, Medicaid's funding is split between each state and the federal government. Medicaid goes by different names in different states (Medi-Cal, Title XIX, Tenncare etc.), which makes this a bit confusing. To find out more information about Medicaid in your state, contact your state Department of Social Services, Welfare, Social Security, or Office of Health Plans (even here, the state-to-state variability of who oversees Medicaid is significant.)

What does Medicaid pay for?

Each state is able to set guidelines—within federally defined parameters—for who is eligible and what services will be covered under the Medicaid benefit. In most states, Medicaid covers a broad array of services, which include inpatient and outpatient care, medication assistance, home health care services, laboratory tests, vaccines, and long-term nursing home care.

For people who are eligible for both Medicare and Medicaid, medications will be covered through Medicare D. And for some Medicare beneficiaries—whose income and assets fall below a specified level—Medicaid will also pick up the co-pays and premiums for Medicare.

How does someone become eligible for Medicaid?

In order to qualify for Medicaid, the person who is ill must meet the eligibility requirements. This will include having a yearly income that falls below a set level, as well as needing to have assets (bank accounts, stocks, mutual funds, property, etc.) that are less than a specified amount. Because Medicaid is funded in part at the state level, and not exclusively at the federal level like Medicare, it will be important to get the rules that are specific to your state.

Resources that can help you determine if you are eligible include:

- Your state's Department of Social Services/Department of Health and Human Services, or a similar agency
- Centers for Medicare and Medicaid (CMS); here is a general link on the topic of eligibility: http://www.cms.hhs.gov/MedicaidEligibility

If you believe that you or your loved one are eligible, the next step is to complete the application and submit it to your local Department of Social Services. Even if you're not certain, starting the application process and having a case worker assigned to help you should help clarify the rules that will pertain to your particular situation. You might even want to consider hiring an attorney with expertise in Medicaid law, if this is a financially viable option. This strategy will help you clarify the rules that pertain to your state and will hopefully avoid a denial of benefits and a large nursing home bill.

What is a Medicaid spend-down?

A Medicaid spend-down refers to the process by which a person reduces their personal assets and income to meet Medicaid requirements in their state. For people with Alzheimer's and dementia who require residential or extensive in-home care, an income spend-down often happens naturally with the accumulation of medical bills.

Will my mom lose the house if Dad has to go onto Medicaid?

The well spouse is able to stay in the family home regardless of its value, as long as she lives in it at the time the application is processed. This question speaks to a real fear that many people have regarding Medicaid—that the well spouse will also need to spend down all of their assets so that the person with dementia can have Medicaid pay for their long-term care. To prevent this spousal impoverishment from happening, there are provisions in the Medicaid Act that allow the well husband or wife to have some resources to remain in the community, and hopefully at or near their previous standard of living.

What other assets can Dad keep if Mom is on Medicaid and in a nursing home?

In addition to the home, the well spouse is able to keep one car, half of the couple's assets, burial funds, and some other specified items. However, there are federally set limits on the maximum and minimum amounts of assets the well spouse can keep—this is called the Community Spouse Resource Allowance or Protected Resource Amount. These amounts are adjusted every January and are currently set at a minimum of $20,880 and a maximum of $104,000. The well spouse's income will not be included in the calculation of assets. However, there is state-to-state variability that impacts the rules, so contacting your particular state's Department of Social Services, an equivalent agency, or an elder law attorney is important.

Chapter 13

ADVANCE DIRECTIVES

- What are advance directives?
- At what point should someone with a dementia make plans for the future?
- What is a power of attorney?
- Are there different types of power of attorney?
- What is a living will?
- What is a health care decision-maker or health care proxy?
- What is a trust fund?
- Why would a person with dementia and their caregiver(s) want to set up a trust?
- Who is qualified to set up a trust?
- Can trusts shelter assets from Medicaid if a person goes into a nursing home?
- What is long-term health insurance?
- What are comfort measures?
- What is a DNR order?
- What happens if someone does not have a DNR order?
- What is hospice care?
- How does someone with dementia become eligible for hospice care?
- How can I ensure that my advance directives will be followed?

What are advance directives?

My physician just told me that I'm having problems with my memory. I could see her struggle with giving me the actual diagnosis. So I asked her straight out, "Is it Alzheimer's?"

She said, "I can't rule that out." And she gave me medication that she said, "will slow things down a little."

What scares me most is that it's always been important for me to feel in control. Now, I try to see the future and I worry about so many things. I picture my children—who, even now that they're adults and have their own families still fight like cats and dogs—fighting tooth and nail over 'what to do with Dad.'

Worse, I worry about my wife getting burdened with all the responsibilities I've always taken care of, not to mention her own health problems. Then there's the question of money—will our savings hold out? What happens if I need to go into a home?

I want to be able to make my own decisions and have them stick. And when I get really sick, I don't want to wind up in a hospital hooked up to a lot of tubes, I just want to be free from pain and treated with some dignity.

Among the challenges of having or caring for someone with dementia are the many legal, financial, medical, and even philosophical and spiritual decisions that need to be thought through. "Advance directives" is a broad term that describes decisions and legal strategies you make while healthy, that legally tell others what you want, should you no longer be able to do so. Advance directives can pertain to all dimensions of a person's life and eventual death. This includes financial planning, residential planning, and what kinds of health care decisions you want made, should you not be able to make your wishes known at that time.

Typical advance directive strategies (all of which we'll discuss individually) can include:

- Appointment of a health care decision-maker/power of attorney for health care or proxy (depending on the state you live in, these go by slightly different names)
- Power of attorney
- Living will; this will likely include end-of-life directions for health care providers
- Trusts (typically not considered an advance directive, but a useful tool for seeing that your wishes are followed regarding money and/or assets)
- Wills—while not traditionally considered a part of advance directives, an up-to-date will is one of the documents you'll want to have completed while you are still healthy.

An attorney with experience in elder law will be able to talk you through the specifics of advance directives. In addition there are a number of excellent resources that include:

- The American Bar Association's "Consumer's Tool kit for Health Care Advance Planning" is available by mail, phone order, or online.
  740 15th Street NW, Washington, DC 20005–1019
  Tel: 202–662–1000
  Website: http://www.abanet.org/aging/toolkit/home.html
- The American Association of Retired Persons (AARP), www.aarp.org
- The National Hospice and Palliative Care Organization offers an excellent state-by-state resource for advance directives, including forms, http://www.caringinfo.org/stateaddownload
- The National Academy of Elder Law Attorneys (NAELA), www.naela.org

At what point should someone with a dementia make plans for the future?

It is best to draft and execute any legal documents as soon as possible once a diagnosis of early dementia or mild cognitive impairment has been made. Even for people with no illness whatsoever, setting up advance directives is a smart idea. Thinking through your preferences and what medical and financial decisions you would like made if you're no longer able to do so helps preserve autonomy and ensures that decisions around your care and well-being will be made in a manner you would want.

It is best to find an attorney who is well-versed or specializes in elder law as soon as possible. Once the dementia has progressed beyond the mildest stage, it becomes more complicated—was the person really competent to sign that document? Will it hold up if challenged?

One suggestion your attorney may make, regardless of the stage of dementia, is to have a psychiatric or psychological evaluation that addresses different areas of judgment and decision-making ability. This will record and prove your level of ability at the time documents were signed, and hopefully decrease any risk that they will be later challenged. Areas covered in this evaluation will likely include:

- Finances
  - Does the person understand what they own?
  - Do they have a general, and realistic, understanding of money coming in and the monthly bills?
  - Can they perform simple arithmetic, as would be required in keeping a checkbook or reconciling a bank statement?
- Medical
  - Are they aware of their current medical condition?
  - Are they able to express reasonable desires around what types of care they do and do not want?

◆ Do they understand the consequences of refusing life-saving treatment if they are seriously ill?

This evaluation will help demonstrate what abilities were still functioning at the time the documents—a will, power of attorney, medical decision-maker, etc.—were drawn up and signed.

What is a power of attorney?

A power of attorney is a legal document that gives another person (referred to as the agent or attorney-in-fact) the authority to make specific legal decisions for the person who signed it (the principal). Unlike a guardianship or conservatorship (discussed in the next chapter), a power of attorney is drawn up when the person with dementia is still able to make their own decisions. Another major difference is that guardians and conservators must report back to the court as a monitoring measure; this is not the case with a power of attorney.

The document can be broad and cover all decisions, or it might be quite specific about what kinds of decisions may be made by the attorney in fact—financial, housing, or legal issues such as any litigation. Decisions around health care are typically not part of this type of power of attorney, but instead are covered under what is called a health care power of attorney, health care proxy, or health care decision-maker (discussed on page 181).

Having a power of attorney for a person with dementia can be an extremely useful strategy to keep things running smoothly. Typical things that an agent or attorney-in-fact is able to do include:
- Pay bills, mortgage payments, utilities, etc.
- Handle banking
- Sign tax returns
- Handle property transactions
- Provide for maintenance to a home

Are there different types of power of attorney?

There are three major types of power of attorney: durable, nondurable, and springing.

- Durable power of attorney. This type of power of attorney begins once it is signed and continues even after the person who signed it is no longer mentally able to make their own decisions. It stays in effect until death, or until the person who signed it decides to revoke it.
- Nondurable power of attorney. This is either a time- or function-limited power of attorney. It might be used if someone were going on vacation and needed someone else to sign a legal document on their behalf. It ends at the point that the person who the agreement concerns becomes disabled or is deemed incompetent by a judge. In general this would not be the type of power of attorney someone with dementia would want.
- Springing power of attorney. Here the word "springing" means that the document goes into effect at some point in the future. In the case of dementia, it could be when the person is no longer able to make reasonable decisions on their own behalf.

For caregivers and people with dementia it is most likely that you will want either a durable power of attorney, or in the case of mild cognitive impairment or very early dementia, you may opt for a springing power of attorney.

What is a living will?

Living wills are documents that provide guidance to health care providers, as well as to your friends and family, about what kinds of medical treatment you would want—or not want—should you no longer be able to communicate your wishes. A living will is a way of letting people know what your wishes are should you be faced with an incurable or end-stage illness. For many this will involve specifically stating whether or not you want aggressive medical measures taken should there be no realistic chance of recovering from the condition.

Directions in a living will can include the withholding or removing of life-sustaining treatment, such as the use of feeding tubes, antibiotics, or even cardio-pulmonary resuscitation should you stop breathing and/or go into cardiac arrest.

What is a health care decision-maker or health care proxy?

As a part of your advance directives you will want to draw up a legal document and appoint someone who can make health care decisions for you if you are unable to do so, either as a result of dementia or in an emergency situation. This can be a relative or friend whom you trust to speak on your behalf.

In choosing your health care decision-maker or proxy, you need to consider a number of factors:

- Is this person willing to take on this responsibility? Not just now, but for the long run?
- Is this someone who shares your values, especially about the kinds of medical treatment you would or would not want?
- Is this someone who is able to speak up for you, even if it might involve conflict with other family members or health care providers?
- Is this someone who has the time to do this, and can they be easily reached in an emergency?
- Do they live nearby, and could they come to a hospital or other health care facility if necessary?
- Is this someone who is legally able to do this? States may exclude certain people, such as those who are not eighteen or

people directly involved in providing your health care, such as your doctor.

What is a trust fund?

A trust fund is an arrangement in which property owned by one person (the owner) is managed by another (the manager or trustee) for the benefit of a third (the beneficiary). In the case of a person with dementia it is possible that they will be both the owner and the beneficiary, and someone else will manage the property. The property refers to any kind of asset the person wants to put into a trust; this could be a home, a business, bank accounts, stocks, bonds, etc.

There are many different types of trusts, including ones that transfer ownership of the property at the time of the beneficiary's death. All true trusts are overseen by trust instruments, which outline who the beneficiaries are, who gets the property when the trust terminates (all trusts must have a termination plan), how money may be distributed among the beneficiaries, who the trustees are, and what are their duties and powers.

In general, in order to set up a trust, the owner must fully understand what they are signing. As this relates to dementia, if a trust is being considered it must be completed when the person is still in the earliest stages of the illness and is determined to have the capacity to sign such a document.

Why would a person with dementia and their caregiver(s) want to set up a trust?

A well-crafted trust removes control of the asset from the person with dementia and gives it firmly to the person managing the trust. This manager or "trustee" then has the ability to use the assets of the trust to provide for the health and well-being of the person with dementia. The trust is able to pay for many important expenses, everything from health insurance, long-term care insurance, doctors, hospitals, and even regular birthday presents to grandchildren.

A trust is often drafted in addition to a power of attorney because there are certain things that cannot be managed through a trust or paid into a trust, such as Social Security and pensions. Likewise, the signing of income tax returns cannot be done through a trust, but could be done with a person's power of attorney.

Who is qualified to set up a trust?

Generally this is done by an attorney, and it's important that the lawyer you select is experienced in estate planning. You might want to look for an attorney who is a member of the National Association of Estate Planners and Councils. You can find such an attorney by contacting:

National Association of Estate Planners and Councils
1120 Chester Ave., Suite 470, Cleveland, OH 44114
Tel: 216–696–3225
Website: www.naepc.org

While it is legal for you to draft and execute a trust on your own—and there are legal software packages out there that can help—based on the potential complexity of trusts it is strongly advised that you get assistance from a professional.

Can trusts shelter assets from Medicaid if a person goes into a nursing home?

No; it is illegal to fund a trust with the purpose of hiding assets from Medicaid. There are complex rules about what assets a person can have or cannot have to qualify for Medicaid.

However, it may be possible for an individual to fund a trust and still be eligible for Medicaid at a later date (five years and one month for certain trusts), or even immediately with certain trusts for disabled children. You will likely want to consult a lawyer who has experience with Medicaid to see what you can legally put in trust.

What is long-term health insurance?

Long-term health insurance policies are purchased when people are well and are there in case someone later needs care, or ongoing placement, in an extended-care facility such as a nursing home. Policies may also cover other ongoing services, such as in-home care, adult day care, and in some cases it can even help pay for an assisted-living facility. Policies may also cover respite care, either in a facility or in the home.

Long-term care insurance is separate from the limited rehabilitation coverage people get with Medicare A, or the long-term coverage people on Medicaid receive. One reason people purchase long-term care insurance is that they want some reassurance that, should they need home care or nursing home placement, they will not have to use up their assets and be subjected to the complex and ever-changing rules around Medicaid.

Many insurance companies offer long-term care policies. There is no standard as to what the benefits are, so understanding what a policy does and does not cover is important. You'll want to understand what the policy will pay on a daily basis, as well as whether or not there is a maximum amount the policy will pay out over the course of a person's lifetime. Things to keep in mind in selecting a policy include:

- What is the cost of the monthly or yearly premiums—these will vary based on the level of coverage, the deductible, and the age at which you enroll (typically the younger you are the lower the premium).
- How long will the benefits last—will it cover one year in a nursing home? Three? Five? Or does it have a lifetime benefit?

- How much will the policy cover for different services on a daily, weekly, or monthly basis?
- Does the policy make allowances for inflation? Many policies will offer inflation protection for an added cost.
- What is the deductible? In long-term care plans, this is some-times called a "waiting period." This is the amount of time you're receiving a service—such as the number of days in a nursing home—before the policy begins to pay.
- What percentage of different services will the policy cover? Do they pay 100 percent or will there be co-pays?
- Do you have to keep paying the premium when you are receiving benefits?

Some employers, as a part of their benefits package, may offer long-term insurance, or do so at a reduced rate with monthly or weekly pre-tax deductions taken from your paycheck. For more information on long-term care insurance, the following organizations can help:

- Area Agency on Aging
  Tel: 800–677–1116 (national number)
  Website: www.n4a.org (national association)
- The American Association of Retired Persons (AARP)
  601 E Street NW, Washington, DC 20049
  Tel: 888–687–2277
  Website: www.aarp.org/money/financial_planning/financial_insurance/a2002–08–13-InsuranceLongTermCare.html
- American Health Care Association
  1201 L Street NW, Washington, DC 20005
  Tel: 202–842–4444
  Website: www.ahcancal.org

What are comfort measures?

Comfort measures are an approach of treatment used in people who have terminal illnesses—such as late Alzheimer's—who have decided that they no longer want invasive procedures or resuscitation should they stop breathing or go into cardiac arrest. It is common for people to spell out in their living will what kind of measures they do or do not want taken in the event of end-stage disease. These can be quite specific, including whether you'd want antibiotics or even a feeding tube. The goal with comfort is not to prolong life, but to keep the person as comfortable as possible—if you are in pain, that is treated.

What is a DNR order?

DNR, which stands for "do not resuscitate," is a directive for health care providers to not attempt CPR or put your loved one on a breathing machine should they stop breathing or go into cardiac arrest. The decision to declare someone DNR is typically done one of two ways. In the first, the individual with dementia can have earlier made her wishes known and formally put these into writing with her advance directives.

If this has not been done, whenever someone is admitted to a hospital or nursing home, paperwork is completed around advanced directives and whether or not someone is to be resuscitated. If a health care decision-maker has been appointed, she will be asked whether or not her loved one is to be resuscitated. If there is no designated decision-maker, conservator, guardian, etc., then family will be consulted.

What happens if someone does not have a DNR order?

Unless there is a signed DNR order in the medical record, when a person in a convalescent home or hospital stops breathing or goes into cardiac arrest, the medical professionals will perform cardiopulmonary resuscitation (CPR). This includes injecting strong medications to try and restart the heart, and placing a hard-plastic tube down the person's throat so they can be more easily oxygenated through the use of a deflatable bag or breathing machine. If the heart has stopped beating, chest compressions are applied at a rate of approximately one per second.

For people with advanced dementia, the chances that CPR will be effective to where they are able to leave the hospital are almost zero. CPR is not a gentle procedure, especially in a frail person; complications can include broken ribs, bruises, and aspiration pneumonia (stomach contents getting into the lung).

What is hospice care?

Hospice care is for people with terminal illnesses—a life expectancy of six months or less—for whom aggressive medical therapies are no longer possible or desired. The hospice philosophy and goal is to keep people as comfortable as possible as they near the end of their life. Hospice care can be provided in the person's home, in the caregiver's home, or in a facility such as a convalescent home, extended-care facility, or residential hospice.

Hospice care emphasizes managing pain, preserving dignity, and providing emotional, social, and spiritual support to the patient and their family. Because hospice care does not seek to lengthen life through extraordinary medical means, feeding tubes, intravenous fluid replacement, dialysis for kidney failure, and even antibiotics are usually not used. However, aggressive pain management is typically a goal of hospice care.

How does someone with dementia become eligible for hospice care?

A referral to a hospice program can be initiated by a simple phone call to a local hospice. The hospice program will gather the initial information and contact your physician for the formal referral. Alternatively, you could discuss hospice care directly with your physician and request that she initiate the referral. Because hospice care—like other medical care—will be paid for through your insurance, Medicare, Medicaid, or even VA benefits, it will need to be authorized and overseen by a physician.

The following resources and agencies can help answer your questions and even locate programs.

- The Hospice Foundation of America
- Tel: 800–854–3402
- Website: www.hospicefoundation.org
- The National Hospice and Palliative Care Association
- Tel: 800–658–8898
- Spanish help line: 877–658–8896
- Website www.caringinfo.org

How can I ensure that my advance directives will be followed?

Most of us are not thrilled to talk about our own death and what we want in the event of serious or terminal illness. However, to increase the likelihood that your advance directives are followed, there are a number of things you can do. Most important is to discuss your wishes with your family, friends, and health care providers. This communication is vitally important, because in the midst of a medical emergency, if people aren't clear, health care providers are obliged to do everything to sustain life—even if that's not what the person had wanted.

Beyond ensuring that your family, friends, and health care providers know you have drawn up advance directives, there are a number of other strategies that will help see that your wishes are followed:

- Carry a card in your wallet or purse with your advance directives and the name and number of your health care power of attorney (health care decision-maker/health care proxy).
- Make sure your signed and notarized documents can be easily found by family or friends.
- Make sure your health care proxy has a copy of your living will and other advance directive documents.
- Consider giving other family members or friends copies of your advance directives in the event your health care proxy cannot be reached.
- Have your physician place a copy of your advance directives in your medical record.
- If you or your loved one is in an institution such as a nursing home, make sure that a copy of the advance directive is in their chart.
- Some organizations will register living wills, such as the U.S. Living Will Registry.

Chapter 14

OTHER LEGAL AND FINANCIAL ISSUES

- What is an elder law attorney?
- How do I find an elder law attorney that is right for me?
- What kinds of things can an elder law attorney help with?
- What if you can't afford an attorney?
- What is a guardian or conservator?
- What are the different types of guardianship or conservatorship?
- When would someone get a conservator versus a power of attorney?
- Who determines if someone is no longer able to make their own decisions?
- When should someone with dementia have a conservator appointed?
- How do I get my dad a guardian/conservator?
- Can someone with dementia write or rewrite their will?
- Can someone with dementia sign other legal documents?
- What are the laws around "gifting" away assets to get on Medicaid?
- What are elder abuse, mistreatment, and neglect?
- What are the signs of abuse and neglect?
- What do I do if I suspect someone with dementia is being mistreated?

What is an elder law attorney?

Elder law is a relatively new legal subspecialty that focuses on issues of later life. Elder law attorneys should be well-versed in drafting wills and advance directives, as well as guiding their clients through potentially complex issues around taxes, gifting, setting up trusts, and even Medicare and Medicaid. For the person with dementia and their caregivers, an elder law attorney can help plan for the different stages of the illness.

It's important when selecting an attorney to ensure that they are able to handle your particular needs, and to remember that not all attorneys—even those who bill themselves as specialists in elder law—are comfortable and experienced in all aspects of elder law. Remember to get references, and consider checking with your local Bar Association to see if there have been any complaints filed about an attorney before hiring him or her to handle your affairs. Mistakes on the part of your attorney can be costly and both emotionally and financially draining, so make sure you're confident in your decision before committing to working with someone.

How do I find an elder law attorney that is right for me?

Probably the best way to find an attorney with special expertise in elder law is through a referral from someone with firsthand experience of working with that attorney. If you are in the process of having a dementia evaluation, it is likely that the medical professionals you are working with will have a list of local attorneys their patients and caregivers have used in the past with good results. Other local sources of referral might include your state's Legal Services Program (depending on your state, this could also be called Legal Aid Program or something similar), your Area Agency on Aging, or your town's senior services.

The Internet is another source of referrals, and the following websites will provide lists of attorneys who either belong to elder law organizations, or who market themselves as having experience in elder law. Many attorneys and law firms maintain websites where they post biographies that include specializations and experience. Some helpful websites with state-by-state resources include:

- The National Academy of Elder Law Attorneys; directory listing at http://naela.org/Applications/ConsumerDirectory/ index.cfm
- Martindale-Hubbell has an online resource at www.martindale.com. Most attorneys are listed here, together with their specialties, training, and some reviews.
- The Alzheimer's Association, www.alz.org.

Finally, your state Bar Association may be able to give you names of attorneys specializing in elder law.

What kinds of things can an elder law attorney help with?

When you have located prospective attorneys, it's a good idea to get some sense of their expertise in the different aspects of the law that you want addressed. While special certification in elder law is not required, many attorneys have pursued this added credential through the National Academy of Elder Law Attorneys. You'll likely want to know if the attorney in question has experience in:

- Laws around Medicare and Medicaid
- Social security law, including disability insurance and handling disability claims
- Estate planning
- Divestiture (gifting) of property, especially if someone may end up in a nursing home and on Medicaid

- Probate, including guardianships
- All aspects of drafting advance directives
- Laws around abuse, neglect, and mistreatment of elders
- Insurance law
- Trusts
- The rules and laws around nursing homes, life-care facilities, and other residential or institutional settings
    - Advocacy for people in nursing homes and other institutional settings
    - Understanding the rights of residents in extended care
- Contracts for assisted-living, life-care, and extended-care facilities
- Mortgages and reverse mortgages

What if you can't afford an attorney?

In 1975, the Older Americans Act was signed into law. Included in this legislation was the provision for funding legal services to older individuals who couldn't otherwise afford them. To find out whether or not you or your loved one qualify, contact your state's legal aid or legal services office, or your Area Council on Aging.

Additionally, many attorneys do a certain amount of pro bono (free) work. The American Bar Association (ABA) maintains a state-by-state listing of pro bono and public service programs at www.abanet.org/legalservices/probono/directory.html#.

What is a guardian or conservator?

A guardian, also referred to as a conservator in certain states, is a person with the legal authority to make decisions for someone else (the ward), who has been deemed by a court to be no longer competent to do so. The authority is given by a judge, most usually a probate judge of the town or city where the person resides. It is common in the case of dementia for a family member, spouse, or significant other to take on the role of guardian or conservator, although this does not have to be the case. It could be a friend or even a stranger appointed by the court to take on this responsibility.

Guardians and conservators will be required to report periodically to the court, and for those who handle finances, there will need to be evidence of appropriate handling of money and property.

What are the different types of guardianship or conservatorship?

The laws around types of guardianships vary by state. Some states view guardianship as all-or-nothing, which means a person is declared incompetent to make any decisions and someone is appointed to do this for them. Recent trends, in an effort to support autonomy and the rights of the individual, have led more states to specify what kinds of decisions a guardian is able to make. It is increasingly common that a court will appoint a financial conservator (conservator of estate), and another guardian to make other kinds of decisions, including medical decisions and decisions around housing (conservator of person). In states that do break up the guardianship around finance and "person," the court may appoint one individual to do both or two separate individuals, one for each guardianship.

When would someone get a conservator versus a power of attorney?

In order to sign legal documents, a person must have the capacity to understand what it is they are signing. As the ability to comprehend and retain information is lost in Alzheimer's and other progressive dementias, executing legal documents will no longer be possible. In the absence of a previously executed power of attorney, a court must now appoint a guardian(s) or conservator(s) to help make decisions and provide for care.

This question again speaks to the importance of planning ahead. Someone in the early stages of dementia may have the capacity to execute a power of attorney, but six months or a year or two later, they may not.

Who determines if someone is no longer able to make their own decisions?

The final decision to declare someone legally unable to make their own decisions is made by a judge, usually a probate judge. The judge, operating under your state's laws, will require additional documentation and possibly even the testimony and evaluations of others stating why this individual is no longer capable of making reasonable decisions. Frequently they will want input from a physician, often in the form of a psychiatric or psychological evaluation that focuses on the person's ability to reason, and their judgment and understanding of important things going on in their lives, such as:

- Do they understand what is wrong with them medically?
- Do they understand the risks and benefits of having, or refusing, treatment?
- Do they know what they own and how much money they have coming in monthly, as well as the monthly bills?
- Are they able to maintain their safety at home and could they handle an emergency—such as the power going out, or a fire in the building—in a reasonable manner?

If the judge determines that the person can no longer make sound decisions, and no power of attorney has been chosen, the judge will appoint a guardian to manage the person's affairs.

When should someone with dementia have a conservator appointed?

In general, the law protects an individual's right to make their own decisions. There is a general principle of "least restrictive," which means people should be able to decide things for themselves unless it is clearly demonstrated that they are no longer able to do so. Each state will define in law when someone has become so disabled that they are no longer able to care for their basic needs and make their own decisions. A loss of capacity goes beyond just making some bad decisions; it implies that the person is not able to provide for basic needs such as food, clothing, personal safety, and shelter. Examples in a person with dementia might include:

- No longer having adequate food in the home, because they're unable to get through all of the steps involved in shopping or arranging for food delivery
- Bills not being paid, to the point where there is threat of foreclosure/eviction or utilities being turned off
- Refusal or lack of life-saving or life-sustaining medical care because they do not understand the consequences
- Dangerous behaviors as a result of the dementia, such as fires in the home or wandering

Other circumstances in which you may need to pursue guardianship are if the person is being robbed or conned out of their money or is refusing to pay for basic necessities. It is only after a person is deemed incompetent to make their own decisions that a guardian or conservator is able to be appointed.

How do I get my dad a guardian/conservator?

Guardianship, or conservatorship, is done through your state's court system—typically through probate court. An application is filed with the court by a family member, friend, health care provider, or even by an agency, such as adult protective services, or the area council on aging.

As part of this application you will need to have one or more physicians—often a psychiatrist—give a sworn statement (affidavit) or testify in person that the person is not able to make reasonable judgments. It will be up to the judge to make the determination as to whether or not a guardian or conservator is to be appointed.

Can someone with dementia write or rewrite their will?

Whether or not a person diagnosed with dementia can write or rewrite a will depends on a few things:

- They need to know what it is they're doing. Do they understand that they are writing a will that will distribute their belongings after they have died?
- They need to know what they own—their assets and belongings.
- They need to understand who their heirs are—family (children, grandchildren), friends, and other beneficiaries of their estate such as charitable organizations.
- They need to understand how they are dividing up their property

Even if the above are met, it's common for an attorney drawing up a will for a person with dementia to request a psychiatric or psychological evaluation to help document that the person was able to understand the basics. Down the road, if the will is questioned or contested, this evaluation will help prove that the person did in fact meet the standard of competence needed to write/rewrite a will (testamentary capacity).

Can someone with dementia sign other legal documents?

Like a will, signing legal documents is dependant upon a person's capacity as to what they are, and are not, still able to do. In legal terms, capacity refers to a person's ability to understand what it is they are doing and the consequences of their choices. Once someone is no longer able to weigh the general pros and cons of a choice, they can no longer sign legal documents, give permission for health care, or transfer property or other assets.

Since the majority of dementia is progressive, this issue of capacity speaks to the importance of taking care of legal affairs as soon as possible in the course of the illness. Also, capacity is not an all-or-nothing issue, especially in the early stages of dementia or with people who have mild cognitive impairment (MCI). A question that is often raised is "capacity for what?" A person with dementia might still be able to make reasonable decisions in one area of their life, but not in others.

Also, different legal documents may not require as high a degree of understanding as others. Drafting a will may still be okay with someone with a mild or even early to moderate degree of dementia if the person understands—in a general way—the issues laid out in the previous question. However, as we head into more specific and complex documents, the degree of understanding needs to be higher. A power of attorney that will give over control of assets and bank accounts to another individual while the person is still alive requires more preserved capacity. Higher still would be the signing of a trust, contracts, or property transfers. You do not want someone with dementia to make legal decisions they don't understand; proceed with caution and only allow them to do that which they are capable of doing.

What are the laws around "gifting" away assets to get on Medicaid?

In 1996, a health insurance reform act was passed—often referred to as the Kennedy-Kassebaum Bill—which, among its various parts, includes rules prohibiting the "gifting" of assets with the purpose of spending down to meet Medicaid eligibility. These rules have been revised a number of times, most recently on February 8, 2006, through the Deficit Reduction Act. Boiled down, what the law says is that transferring any property for less than its "fair market value" will be considered an attempt to fraudulently meet Medicaid eligibility. Any gifts made within a five-year "look-back" period before filing a Medicaid application will be subject to penalties. Prior to the 2006 change, the look-back period was three years. All gifts, no matter how small, are subject to this look-back, so even gifts to charities and religious organizations can be reviewed and a penalty applied.

The penalty takes the form of days, weeks, months, or even years tacked onto the amount of time before someone can be eligible for Medicaid. So if you apply today, but have given away property and cash within the look-back period, you will not be eligible for Medicaid until the time has elapsed that equals the amount of money you have given away divided by the daily cost of nursing home care ($100/day, $3,000/month). So if you gave away $10,000, that would equal 100 days.

Also remember that, while some of the rules/laws are made at the federal level, there may be some state-to-state differences. Understanding the exact rules in your state is important.

What are elder abuse, mistreatment, and neglect?

- *"I just went to see Mom at the home, and she was sitting in front of her meal tray and no one was feeding her. Don't they know she won't eat unless someone helps her?"*

- *"I got a look inside the condo of the man living next door. It doesn't look like he's cleaned in months and there is garbage piled every-where. His children moved him into the retirement community five months ago; I think something's wrong."*
- *"Mom just told me that she's been giving her jewelry to her aide. I told her to stop, but she's beyond the point where she'll even remember."*
- *"I asked the nurse why Mom is such a zombie today. They've been giving her tranquilizers every time she has an outburst. I know that's not what the doctor recommended."*

Elder abuse, mistreatment, and neglect are terms that describe either deliberate or unintended ways in which caregivers—or others upon whom an older person relies—cause them harm or put them in harm's way. Elder abuse includes older people with dementia who may have no formal or informal caregivers and who are no longer able to care for themselves (self-neglect). The abuse and neglect can come in many different forms:

- Physical
  - Assault
  - Use of restraints—both physical and chemical
  - Sexual assault
  - Overmedication/under medication/lack of medication super-vision in someone who is unable to manage it themselves
  - Denial of needed medical care
- Emotional/psychological
  - Coercion and threats
  - Shouting or screaming at the person with dementia
- Financial
  - Theft of money and property
  - Embezzlement
- Deprival of basic needs

- Inadequate food in the home
- Utilities disconnected
- Unsanitary living conditions
- Unsafe housing

What are the signs of abuse and neglect?

Because elder abuse and neglect can occur in so many ways, being alert for signs that someone is being mistreated or unable to provide for their own care is important. This is especially true for people with more advanced dementia who may not be able to communicate what is happening to them.

Physical signs of abuse can include:

- Bruises, including signs that the person has been forcibly restrained or choked
- Fractures and dislocations
- Signs of medical neglect such as bed sores or contractures, a permanent condition in which the person's muscles and ligaments deteriorate as a result of inadequate movement
- Abnormal findings on blood work that might indicate the person has been over- or under-medicated or deprived of basic nutrition and hydration
- Torn clothing or broken dentures or glasses
- The use of physical or chemical restraints, including using tranquilizers and sedating medications to keep the person quiet

Signs of neglect may include:

- Poor hygiene, clothing that is not clean, lack of adequate bathing
- Someone being locked inside their house when no caregiver is there
- Being left unattended inside a car

- Inadequate heating and cooling
- Weight loss

Emotional signs of neglect and abuse may include:
- Any reports by the older person that they are being abused should be investigated
- Changes in behavior, often with an increase in anxiety and fear
- For someone with an advanced dementia, the behavioral change may involve tantrums, rocking, thumb sucking, or head banging
- Relatives or caregivers refusing to allow health care providers, other family members, or friends from having access to the individual
- Caregivers have been observed yelling at or being mean and derogatory to the older person

Financial signs of abuse may include:
- Unexplained withdrawals from bank accounts, signing over deeds, securities, etc.
- The person not having adequate funds to meet their usual expenses

Signs of self-neglect may include:
- The person living in unhealthy or filthy conditions
- The person continuing to live in housing that is neglected and unsafe
- Utilities being turned off
- Lack of adequate food
- The person behaving in bizarre, erratic, or dangerous ways, such as barricading doors and windows, shouting or screaming, setting fires—either intentionally or not—or wandering from the home

What do I do if I suspect someone with dementia is being mistreated?

All states have laws concerning what to do if you suspect that an older person is being mistreated or abused. Most states require health care professionals to report any suspected cases of abuse, and may even fine them if they don't. Regardless of the law, if you suspect that an older person is being mistreated or not caring for themselves adequately, it needs to be reported.

In an emergency situation, in which you believe the person is at severe risk of harm and/or needs immediate help, call 911 or your local police. For everything else you can contact your state's office of Adult Protective Services and make a report. Each state has a long-term care ombudsman program, which will investigate all complaints of elder abuse/neglect in long-term care facilities that they receive (this is discussed further in Chapter 15).

A good resource to contact is the National Center on Elder Abuse, which provides state-by-state information. Their address is

1201 15th Street NW, Suite 350, Washington, DC 20005–2842

Tel: 202–898–2586

Fax 202–898–2583

Email: ncea@nasua.org

A state-by-state elder abuse agency locator is available on their website at: http://www.elderabusecenter.org/default.cfm?p= statehotlines.cfm. They also maintain a toll free number for reporting suspected abuse at 1–800–677–1116.

Chapter 15

NURSING HOMES AND EXTENDED-CARE FACILITIES

- How do I know if my dad needs to go into a nursing home?
- How do I know what level of care is right for my mom?
- What is a rest home and how is it different from a nursing home?
- What is an assisted-living facility?
- What is a life-care facility?
- What is a nursing home?
- What does extended-care mean?
- What things should I look for in a nursing home?
- How can I find a good nursing home?
- At what point should I put my husband's name on a nursing home waiting list?
- How can I be sure my mom is getting good care?
- How can I ease the transition to a nursing home?
- Who oversees nursing homes?
- What are my rights in a long-term facility?
- What is a long-term care ombudsman?
- What should I do if I suspect my husband is being mistreated?
- What is an Alzheimer's or dementia unit?
- Is an Alzheimer's unit in an assisted-living facility the same as in a nursing home?

How do I know if my dad needs to go into a nursing home?

The decision to place your loved one in a nursing home is highly individual. What often decides the matter is when you are no longer able to provide and/or arrange for in-home care that is adequate to meet the person's needs. Reasons for the decision to place someone in an extended-care facility or skilled nursing facility include:

- The person is having behavioral symptoms that are more than you can handle—wandering, aggression, loss of bladder or bowel control, inappropriate sexual behavior in a house with children.
- The demands and needs of the rest of your family make it impossible to provide adequate supervision.
- Your own health is not up to the task, and you are jeopardizing your own well-being by continuing to keep the person at home.
- The person requires a level of medical care and/or supervision that you cannot provide.
- You cannot afford the level of in-home care the person needs (round-the-clock aides, in-home nursing not covered by your insurance or Medicare/Medicaid).
- The person is no longer able to negotiate their—or your—home. They can no longer handle stairs, use a tub, etc.

How do I know what level of care is right for my mom?

For most caregivers, the goal in placing a loved one in an extended-care facility is to have a setting where their needs can be safely and consistently met. At the same time, because this will now become the person's home, you don't want them to feel uncomfortable or imprisoned. For people with moderate to severe dementia, you are probably looking for around-the-clock supervision, most likely in a setting where the person is not able to wander off, such as a skilled nursing facility (nursing home).

In situations where the person may be in an earlier stage of dementia, a residential care home, such as a rest home/retirement home or bed and board may be adequate. If there is a need for some medical oversight—but not around-the-clock—an assisted-living facility may be the best fit. Overall, the guiding principal is that you want to leave the person with as much autonomy as is safe and realistic. Beyond this, it's important that the new setting feel as much like home as is possible.

What is a rest home and how is it different from a nursing home?

Rest homes, sometimes called retirement homes, residential care homes, homes for the aged, or bed and board, should not be confused with skilled nursing facilities (nursing homes). In general, people living in rest homes are able to come and go as they please—some of them may request that residents sign in and sign out, but the doors are not locked. Rest homes may help oversee medications, but not all have an on-site nursing staff to administer medications. They do not provide on-site medical care, although many people living in rest homes will be able to have in-home services through a nursing agency, just as if they were in a private residence.

Rest homes typically provide meals and cooking is not allowed in the rooms. Laundry service and housekeeping may also be included. Some will have private rooms, but more typically it's two to a room with a shared bath.

What is an assisted-living facility?

Assisted-living facilities, sometimes called board and care, offer a greater degree of on-site medical care and assistance with ADLs such as bathing and dressing than rest homes do. They differ from nursing homes in that residents will have their own apartments or private rooms with a private or semi-private bath. While they may not offer around-the-clock nursing care, medical assistance is available if needed. Meals are often in a communal setting, such as a dining hall, but the residents are also able to prepare some food in their own kitchenettes. Other available services may include laundry and housekeeping.

Advantages to assisted-living facilities include:

- Socialization in a safe setting. Most will include a variety of activities, communal meals, recreation, etc, that can help diminish feelings of isolation.
- They promote a degree of autonomy and independence. People are able to have their own living space and leave the facility when they want.
- Many assisted-living facilities also offer a separate and secure dementia section, where people are unable to wander off the grounds.

It's important to remember that assisted-living facilities cannot provide the same level of nursing care and supervision found in nursing homes. What this means for someone with a progressive dementia is that assisted-living may be adequate to a point, but should their health or behavior deteriorate they will not be allowed to remain in that facility. So it's important to have a backup plan, such as having the person's name on waiting lists to nursing homes that you both find acceptable.

What is a life-care facility?

Life-care facilities are a relatively new alternative to nursing homes. These are facilities where you buy your own apartment and then pay a monthly fee. The facility includes a variety of specified services such as meals, housekeeping, and general maintenance. If you should become ill while in a life-care facility, they will be able to provide you with increasing levels of support and assistance in your own unit. Or, if your needs exceed what can be safely provided in your own room or apartment, they have a nursing home level of care to which you will be moved.

Different from most assisted-living facilities where you pay only a monthly fee, life-care facilities involve a substantial buy-in fee; but once you have signed your contract, you are provided a guarantee that you or your loved one will be able to remain in the facility indefinitely. If pursuing this option, you may want to involve an attorney in reviewing the contract. Some life-care facilities may be willing to accept people with early dementia, but many will turn down applications from people they believe to have a progressive dementing illness.

What is a nursing home?

A nursing home—or skilled nursing facility—is an institution that provides around-the-clock care and supervision for people with serious medical disabilities, such as dementia. Most nursing homes are able to offer rehabilitative services (occupational, physical, respiratory, and speech therapy) and will have a range of activities for the residents.

Much of the care in nursing homes is provided by aides and nursing assistants under the supervision of registered nurses (RNs) and licensed practical nurses (LPNs). The facility will have a physician as its medical director, and much/most of the person's medical care will be provided within the home.

Nursing homes are licensed through your state's department of public health or an equivalent agency, and are subject to regular surveys. If they accept Medicare and Medicaid reimbursement they will have additional oversight at both the state and federal levels.

What does extended-care mean?

Extended-care is another term for nursing home or skilled nursing facility (SNF). It's used to refer to medical facilities that are able to offer ongoing care for medical problems, such as are seen following strokes or complex surgeries. Extended-care includes a focus on rehabilitation, with treatment plans that incorporate occupational, physical, and other therapies designed to help the person return to a higher level of functioning.

What things should I look for in a nursing home?

In selecting a nursing home for your loved one, many factors will come into play. This is one of the reasons why visiting various facilities well in advance of needing one is a good idea. This will give you the opportunity to compare and contrast what is available. It's important to remember that even though nursing homes are under tough federal and state regulations, there is a tremendous range of quality.

Things you will want to look at and ask questions about include:
- Philosophy
  - Does the facility embrace a person-centered approach to care?
  - Is the patient Bill of Rights prominently displayed?
  - Is it clear who is in charge, and who to go to if there's a problem?
  - Are families encouraged to participate in treatment and treatment planning?
  - Is there an active resident council—how often does it meet and how much are its recommendations valued and used?

- Is there a family council?
- Is there a family support group?
- Is there any statement as to the facility's commitment to becoming restraint-free?
- The facility itself. Use your five senses.
  - Is it modern? How does it look?
  - Does it appear clean?
  - Does it smell?
  - Are there grab rails in the hallway?
  - Are the rooms attractive? Or does it look and feel like a hospital?
  - Is the nursing station close to the residents' rooms?
  - Does it feel homey?
  - How does the food taste? Ask for a sample and observe a mealtime.
  - Feel the sheets. Are they soft? Are they clean?
  - How noisy is it? Are there a lot of bells going off at the nurses' station? Are other residents loud?
- Location
  - Is it close enough to you?
  - Will other people be able to come and visit, or is too far away?
- Staff
  - Is the staff knowledgeable about dementia and Alzheimer's?
  - Do they use a staffing model that promotes consistency? In other words, will your loved one have different aides every day, or will they have someone assigned to them as their primary person?
  - What kind of training is the staff given about working with people with dementia?
  - What kinds of interventions do staff use with behavioral disturbances?

- The residents
  - ◆ Do they appear to be well-groomed?
  - ◆ Are people lying in their beds in the middle of the day?
  - ◆ Do they seem happy?
  - ◆ Are people being restrained or in any way having their freedom of movement restricted by posey vests (a garment that ties a person to their chair or bed) or other means?
- Programming
  - ◆ What activities are offered on a daily basis?
  - ◆ Are there places for people to safely wander?
- Medical oversight
  - ◆ How many nurses are there to a unit? How many aides?
  - ◆ How often will the doctor or APRN see your loved one?
  - ◆ Who is the facility's medical director? And how do they handle medical emergencies?

Most important is choosing a nursing home that both you and your loved one feel comfortable and safe in.

How can I find a good nursing home?

Selecting a nursing home is best done before you find yourself in a crisis and you need one right away. There are many people and organizations who can help you find a good fit. If you've been through a dementia evaluation, ask the staff for recommendations. Likewise, your physician or APRN may be able to steer you to a facility where they would be comfortable having their own family member. Attend a local Alzheimer's Association support group and find out what local nursing homes other people in the same situation have found that meet the needs of the person with dementia and their family. Your local Area Council on Aging is another possible source of referral.

It's important to visit prospective facilities where you can have all of your questions answered. Call and schedule tours at each facility that's been recommended to you.

Some websites and organizations that can help you in your search include:

- **Medicare Nursing Home Compare website**
  This is a very useful online search tool that allows you to do a side-by-side comparison of all nursing homes in a specified geographic area.
  www.medicare.gov/NHCompare

- **National Citizen's Coalition for Nursing Home Reform (NCCNHR)**
  This is an important non-profit organization that advocates for nursing home residents and their families. Their site is filled with useful information that runs the range from what to look for in a nursing home to how to advocate for good care. Their site also contains links for state-by-state information on nursing homes.
  www.nccnhr.org

- **The Alzheimer's Association**
  The Alzheimer's Association maintains an information-packed website that includes a state-by-state locator of services in your area.
  www.alz.org

At what point should I put my husband's name on a nursing home waiting list?

Even during the early stages of Alzheimer's, it's important to think ahead and have a variety of "what if" contingency plans. While your initial intent may be to keep your loved one at home regardless of what happens, for various reasons this is not always possible. Therefore, it's a good idea to ask for recommendations for nursing homes in your area soon after a diagnosis. You'll want to visit, and if you believe that you have found a place where your loved one would be well-cared for and comfortable, go ahead and get their name put on the waiting list. You may want to do this with a number of facilities. Here's why:

- Nursing homes in general may have long waiting lists—some could be years long. This is especially true for facilities that offer specialized Alzheimer's units or have better reputations.
- Putting your loved one's name on a waiting list carries no obligation. If their name comes up, and they don't need that level of care, just turn down the opening and have their name put back on the list. It's important to clearly request that their name remain on the list, and that it's not to come off unless you ask.

How can I be sure my mom is getting good care?

The most important thing you can do is to stay present and involved once you have admitted someone to a nursing home. You need to let the staff know that you are still very involved with the care of your loved one; the best way to do this is through your actions. Do not feel like you are imposing. After all, people with more advanced dementia are not able to consistently and effectively speak up for themselves, or even let others know what their needs are. You know your loved one best, and in this new environment the staff will have to consult with you to help them get their patient's needs met.

- Visit frequently, and at different times of day.
- Participate in treatment planning meetings. These should occur at least every three months.

- Participate in the family council and/or family support groups.
- Observe how staff handles meal times, bath times, and any dressing changes.
- Check to make sure that the medications are correct. If there have been changes that you were not aware of—especially if you are the conservator, medical decision-maker, or guardian—contact the physician who ordered them to find out why the changes were made.
- Make sure that the daily schedule includes adequate physical activities.
- Be alert for any physical signs of poor care, including dehydration, weight loss, bed sores, or muscle contractures (a state in which the muscles constrict and limbs assume a curled-up position due to lack of movement).
- If you have concerns about the care, raise them to the shift supervisor. If you don't feel they are listened to, go higher in the organization. If they are serious concerns and you don't feel they are being adequately addressed by the home, contact your long-term-care ombudsman (see question on ombudsman on page 219) or report your concerns to the state agency that oversees and licenses the facility.

How can I ease the transition to a nursing home?

- *"When I even mention a nursing home, my mother becomes furious and screams at me."*
- *"My dad accuses me of stealing his home; why doesn't he realize it had to be sold to pay for his care and so he could eventually go on Medicaid?"*
- *"Ever since I had my wife admitted to the nursing home, she won't even talk to me."*

Studies looking at the major times of stress in our lives consistently show that any sort of move can be traumatic. This becomes even more of a stress when the move is not something we wanted, and this is often the case when a person with dementia must move from their own home—or your home—into an assisted-living facility or nursing home. Stress can also result from moving in with another family member or caregiver.

Among the losses the person with dementia may experience is the loss of independence, the loss of material possessions, and the loss of surroundings that are familiar—it may be this last issue that is the most potent. While there is no way to eliminate the sometimes harsh reality of these moves, there are many things you can do to ease the transition.

- Bring items from home to decorate the person's new space. Family photos, a favorite afghan and pillows, and other items will bring a sense of the familiar to the new surroundings. If the person has a private room, you might arrange the furniture to replicate their previous bedroom.

- Spend time with the person while they are getting adjusted to the new space. Try not to overwhelm them with doing too much at once.

- Introduce yourself to the staff that will be working with your family member or loved one. Let them know you want to be contacted if there are problems or if they have any concerns.

- Get familiar with the routines of the new facility so that you know what your loved one's day consists of.
  - Learn the daily schedule.
  - If your loved one has special needs, habits, or routines, make sure staff are aware of these and that they get worked into the treatment plan.
  - See how meals are handled—be present for a number of meals to make sure that your loved one is able to handle the routine.

◆ Find out what activities are available to residents, and make sure that these are a part of the schedule. Make a point of attending them with your loved one—especially early in the placement—both to see what is being offered and to let staff know how important keeping your loved one active and interested is to you.

• Put up signs that will help the person with dementia find their way around. Many facilities will put signs on the doors with the person's name. If there is a door on the person's bathroom you might hang a sign that says "Bathroom" or "Kate's Bathroom."

Who oversees nursing homes?

There are multiple levels of oversight for nursing homes and extended-care facilities. They should be licensed by your state's Department of Health or an equivalent agency, and as such they are subject to on-site inspection and review. Because nursing homes bill Medicare and Medicaid, they are subject to the policies and regulations as put forward by the Centers for Medicare and Medicaid. This can include on-site inspections.

Concerns about care need to be addressed. If these cannot be handled by the facility staff and administration, each state has a long-term care ombudsman (see Appendix D) who investigates complaints and works toward getting them resolved.

What are my rights in a long-term facility?

As a resident in either an extended-care facility or a skilled nursing facility, you have many rights and these need to be explained to you and your caregiver(s). Typically these will be posted in easily accessed areas of your facility. They will be titled "Resident's Bill of Rights" or something similar. In addition, you should receive a copy of these at the time of admission.

First and foremost, you are a citizen of the United States and you retain the rights guaranteed to you because of this when you enter an extended-care facility. Among your rights as a patient are:

- A listing of services available to you in the facility
- Your rights and the policies around transfer, discharge, and holding your bed should you need to go to a hospital for any treatment
- Information on administration of medication and whether or not you can administer your own
- The right to refuse treatment or services
- The right to access information about inspections of the facility, including those performed by your state's Department of Public Health or equivalent agency
- The procedure on how to file a complaint or grievance
- Contact information for your state's and region's long-term care ombudsman (see next question)
- Contact information for advocacy groups and elder protective services
- The right to be free from retaliation or other negative consequence should you file a grievance against the facility
- The right to access your records
- The right to participate meaningfully in the creation of your treatment plan
- The right to have visitors
- The right to contact and have access to your care providers, including your physician
- The right to be free from chemical or physical restraints
- The right to be free from any form of abuse (physical, verbal, emotional, sexual, or financial exploitation)
- The right to privacy, including on the telephone and being able to meet privately with visitors

- The right to practice the faith of your choice
- The right to have a daily schedule of your own choosing
- The right to live in a clean and comfortable facility
- The right to manage your own finances
- The right to receive your mail unopened

The above list is not exhaustive, and there will be some differences in what will be in a particular facility's resident's bill of rights. In general, state laws will govern what must be included in the resident's bill of rights.

What is a long-term care ombudsman?

Each state, under the Older Americans Act, has a long-term care ombudsman program. The ombudsman serves as an advocate for people in nursing homes, assisted-living facilities, and retirement homes. The ombudsman can assist in locating nursing homes and assisted-living facilities as well as in helping to resolve conflicts when they arise.

If you or your loved one are experiencing problems in a nursing home and do not believe you will be able to resolve them by working with staff, the ombudsman can be contacted. She will then—with your permission—be able to participate in working through your particular issues. Typically, this will start with her talking to the resident to get their perspective on the situation, as well as their permission to talk to others. This will be done confidentially. In the case of a person with advanced dementia who is not able to articulate their concern, she will speak with family caregivers.

An ombudsman may be able to get the problem resolved quickly by working with the facility's administrators and/or staff. This might include them actually being present and participating in care-planning meetings at the facility. If the problem is more dire (such as frank abuse and/or neglect), or does not improve, she may involve other agencies and individuals such as your state's department of health, the Center for Medicare and Medicaid, or your state's Attorney General.

Ombudsmen are not paid by the facilities and their services are free. To locate your ombudsman refer to Appendix D.

What should I do if I suspect my husband is being mistreated?

- *"Mom developed bed sores. I thought good nursing care was supposed to prevent that."*
- *"Every time I visit Dad he's so doped up he can barely walk. Why are they doing that?"*

If you believe that your loved one is a victim of abuse, neglect, or bad care in a long-term care facility, it is important to rapidly address this. While you—or they—may have concerns about retaliation if the concerns are reported, the risk of them suffering permanent physical or emotional damage is too great. Depending on the nature of the suspected abuse, there are a number of strategies to pursue. Clearly, if it's something serious you need to take immediate and decisive action; for lesser issues, it may be possible to resolve the matter by addressing the issue with the nursing supervisor or administrator. If you do not get a satisfactory answer you will likely want to contact your state's long-term care ombudsman or department of public health. Information, including phone numbers for the ombudsman and other advocacy agencies and organizations in your state, should be clearly posted in the facility along with the Patients' Bill of Rights.

It's a good idea to keep copies of all documentation around the suspected abuse or neglect. If there are signs of physical abuse, take photos. In some instances you may want to pursue legal council from an attorney that specializes in elder law (see Chapter 14).

What is an Alzheimer's or dementia unit?

Many nursing homes now offer specialized units designed for people with Alzheimer's and other dementing illnesses. While there is no standard or established model for this type of unit, some of the kinds of things you would want to look for in a dementia unit include:

- Staff who have been trained to handle behavioral problems with redirection and non-drug strategies as the first, second, and third-line options
- Locked units to prevent wandering
- A simple layout of the rooms to decrease confusion
- Bathrooms that are easily accessible, and if possible, visible from the resident's bed
- Well-lit units to decrease sundowning and confusion
- An effort to maintain a calm and quiet environment
- Daily activities to promote physical well-being and mental stimulation, and to provide socialization
- Some offer an enclosed outdoor space where people are able to safely walk and get fresh air
- Memory aids to help residents find their rooms—this can include putting their name on the door, or color-coding rooms and bathrooms
- Encouraging the involvement of family and other caregivers in ongoing care and treatment

Is an Alzheimer's unit in an assisted-living facility the same as in a nursing home?

No. There will be important differences between the Alzheimer's special care units found in those nursing homes that have them and those that may be offered, or advertised, through some assisted-living facilities. This can be confusing as you would think all dementia units are—or should be—somewhat similar; they're not.

In general, assisted-living facilities are less restrictive than nursing homes. They are not overseen by the federal government and can be thought of as a halfway point between someone being in their own home and a nursing home. Here are some other important points to keep in mind.

- Assisted-living facilities are typically paid for on a month-to-month basis, and there is no promise that the person can remain there forever; if someone's behavior or medical condition progresses beyond what can safely be handled at the facility they will need to move to a higher level of care, such as a nursing home.
- Assisted-living facilities, where people pay for their own room or apartment, offer a greater degree of independence than nursing homes. The apartment portion of the facility will not be locked and people are able to come and go. In units—or floors—specially designed for people with Alzheimer's, the apartments or rooms may be grouped together and include a safe, enclosed area where people may wander without leaving the facility.
- Most assisted-living facilities do not offer around-the-clock, on-site nursing supervision.
- Assisted-living facilities are typically not covered by Medicaid.

It is common for someone with an early-to-moderate dementia to start in an assisted-living facility, where they can benefit from the higher level of independence and socialization. As the dementia progresses, a nursing home level of care may become necessary.

Chapter 16

CARING FOR THE CAREGIVER

- What are the positives to being a caregiver?
- Since my husband's diagnosis I've been very emotional—is this normal?
- Are caregivers at an increased risk for emotional and health problems?
- What can I do to decrease my chances of having physical and emotional problems?
- How do I know if I'm suffering from clinical depression?
- What can I do to get over my depression?
- How do I learn to accept help from others?
- How do I deal with my anger?
- How important is having a support group?
- Where do I find a support group?
- What is respite care?
- How can I maintain a social life if my husband has dementia?
- I don't want everyone to know that John has Alzheimer's; is this wrong?

What are the positives to being a caregiver?

- *"I know my mom doesn't even remember my name, but I love being able to take care of her and give her back some of the love she gave to us."*
- *"We have a lot of fun together; of course it's not the way it used to be, but it's great to see her smile and to know that the care and attention I give her is better than anything she would get in a nursing home."*
- *"I really like spending this time with Dad. I feel like it's brought us closer, and I find that taking care of him brings out a part of me I didn't know I had."*

While a lot of attention is paid—and rightly so—to topics like caregiver burden, burnout, etc., we don't want to lose sight of the fact that most caregivers derive a great deal of meaning, purpose, and enjoyment from what they do. Taking care of another person, especially when it's someone you love, can be emotionally and spiritually fulfilling. For others, the caregiver role may be a strong part of your value system, and looking after a family member, spouse, or a close friend is a moral or even religious obligation. From a purely practical point of view, there may be financial advantages to providing care instead of paying someone to do it.

For caregivers who have learned how to roll with the ups and downs of dementia, there can be the added benefit of realizing just how competent you can be. You should take a sense of pride and accomplishment in how you've been able to manage and get through the rough spots. The caregiver role, while undeniably challenging, can also be a rich opportunity for personal growth.

Finally, many caregivers find pleasure, and even joy, in spending time taking care of their loved one. You may also find reserves of humor and an ability to express affection within yourself that go a long way toward transforming the caregiver experience into one of laughter and warmth.

Since my husband's diagnosis I've been very emotional—is this normal?

- *"James could not believe that the doctor was right. Sure, his wife was a bit more forgetful, and there had been that fender bender, but Alzheimer's? No way, not his Ellen."*
- *"I know it's not Barrie's fault. He didn't ask to have dementia. But everything we've worked for is gone. All of our plans—we were going to travel, spend time going to visit each of our kids...I'm so mad. I feel like everything inside is one great big knot. I feel so guilty, because I'm mad at Barrie. Why did this have to happen?"*
- *"Maybe the doctor is wrong. Maybe this is just something temporary. God, please let it be anything else, just not this. Please let her be okay."*
- *"Ever since I got the news about John I can't sleep, I can't eat, I'm nervous all the time wondering what's going to happen next. I try not to let him see me cry, but it seems that's all I'm doing."*
- *"I miss the woman I married. I know she's gone, and I don't know this person who took her place."*

Whenever we experience a major loss or setback, there are a number of normal emotional changes we can expect. These were well described by Elisabeth Kübler-Ross in her classic work on grief, *On Death and Dying*. Kübler-Ross asserts that people go through five stages of grief: denial, anger, bargaining, depression, and finally acceptance.

Denial of the illness is common, for both the person with dementia and the caregiver. It can take the form of disagreeing with the diagnosis and trying to minimize the objective data as it piles up around you. Getting through this denial and acknowledging that there is a problem becomes critically important so that proper assessment, treatment, and planning for the future can begin.

Likewise, anger is to be expected. Previously made plans and dreams are suddenly called into question. The anger and hurt you feel are part of being human. We like to feel in control of our own destiny, and a diagnosis of Alzheimer's takes some of that sense of control away.

A stone's throw from anger is depression. For both caregivers and people recently diagnosed with dementia, it is common to see emotional changes that, if they go on long enough, can turn into a clinical depression. These emotional changes include sadness, a numb feeling, loss of energy, changes in sleep and appetite, and feelings of hopelessness and despair. In serious depression people may contemplate, or even commit, suicide.

Attempts to bargain—often with God, sometimes with the doctors—are also to be expected:

- *"Maybe it's not Alzheimer's. Are you sure you've done all the tests?"*
- *"God, if you let Joe be well, I promise to be more charitable."*

Finally, people are able to accept the diagnosis. This doesn't mean you have to like it—you probably don't—but you know it to be a reality. With acceptance comes the possibility of getting on with things. You can now revise plans and look toward a different vision of the future. The importance of acceptance—especially for the caregiver—cannot be stressed enough.

While all of the early stages of grief are normal, it becomes a problem if you get stuck in one and can't move on to a place of acceptance. In this chapter we'll look at issues specific to the caregiver and ways to help you through some of the rough spots.

Are caregivers at an increased risk for emotional and health problems?

Various studies looking at the health of caregivers have shown increased rates of clinical depression, anxiety, and other health problems. Additionally, the chance that someone in a caregiver role will die is as much as 63 percent higher than someone who isn't a caregiver, when all other health factors between the two are even.

It's important to understand that our minds and our bodies are connected. Being stressed out or overburdened, if not alleviated, eventually leads to negative physical and emotional changes. When chronically stressed, we produce more "stress hormones," adrenalin and cortisol, which over time can lead to medical conditions including hypertension, elevated cholesterol, depression, and anxiety. All of these increase our overall risk of coronary artery disease, heart attack, and stroke.

Providing care for someone with dementia introduces a number of different and very real stresses into your life. Depending on your particular situation, these may constitute a small problem or a very large one. Sources of stress that caregivers frequently report include:

- Worry over finances
  - *"Can I keep working?"*
  - *"How will I keep up with the mortgage if I don't work?"*
  - *"If my husband goes into a nursing home, will I lose the house?"*
  - *"I can't afford the medication."*
  - *"I can't afford the co-pays for my doctor."*
- Disruption of sleep, especially if the person being cared for has disrupted sleep patterns
- Health concerns, both for yourself and the person you're caring for
- Worries over being able to provide competent care

- ◆ *"I'm not a nurse; I don't know how to do this."*
- ◆ *"What if I do something wrong?"*
- ◆ *"I feel like I'm hurting him every time I give him a bath."*
- Loneliness and isolation
  - ◆ *"I can't see my friends."*
  - ◆ *"Everyone is too embarrassed to visit."*
  - ◆ *"I don't want people to know my business."*
  - ◆ *"I'm ashamed to ask for help; I should be able to do this myself."*

What can I do to decrease my chances of having physical and emotional problems?

A good approach to decreasing your risk of physical and mental health problems is to identify the things that are stressing you out and look for strategies and interventions that will decrease your burden and enhance your well-being. You might want to write your concerns on a piece of paper, and fill in possible solutions or resources that might help next to each. In a sense, this becomes your own treatment plan.

You may be able to lump some stressors and solutions together. For instance, identifying that respite care (see page 239 for more on respite care) might help you get out to see friends, go to the hairdresser, or go to your own doctor could be an intervention for a number of different problems. Likewise, if you feel that you just don't have enough information about finances, how to get onto Medicaid, paying for medications, etc., then perhaps tracking down a comprehensive geriatric or dementia assessment clinic or team (see Chapter 3) might help you with several of these needs at the same time.

Problem/Need	What I'd like/My goal	Possible Solutions/ Interventions
I can't get a good night's sleep because my husband is up all night and I'm worried that he'll wander out of the house or turn on the stove.	6–8 hours of restful sleep	Read a book on non-medication strategies to improve sleep. Ask the doctor for a sleeping medication for my husband. Put alarms on the doors in case he does get out. Unplug the stove at night. Enroll my loved one in the Medic Alert/Safe Return program through the Alzheimer's Association (see Chapter 10).
I'm horribly depressed. I think things are only going to get worse.	To not be depressed. To see a future for myself.	See a mental health professional for counseling and possibly medication. Join an Alzheimer's/dementia support group. Make sure I get adequate amounts of exercise and sunlight.
I worry about money all the time. I'm frightened that I'll lose the house if my wife has to go into a home.	To not worry about my finances.	See a financial planner. Call my local council on aging or Department of Social Services (DSS) so that I can understand the rules about what property a spouse can own if the other spouse has to go on Medicaid and be placed in a nursing home.

Problem/Need	What I'd like/My goal	Possible Solutions/ Interventions
I can't afford both of our medications.	To be able to have all of our prescriptions filled.	Contact your local council on aging to find out what programs you are eligible for that will help you pay for medications. See if you qualify for special assistance under the Medicare D program (see Chapter 11).
I'm very lonely. I feel like I'm shut up inside all day and can't get out to see friends or family.	To spend time every week with friends and family.	Arrange for some form of regular respite. This could be a sitter in the home (friend, relative, or paid aide) or adult day care.

How do I know if I'm suffering from clinical depression?

At seventy-two, Claire realized that her dreams for retirement had gone up in smoke. Her husband Jim, six years older than she, had started to develop Alzheimer's in his early seventies. At first she had ignored the changes: his uncharacteristic mood swings, the way he'd start a project and then she'd find him doing something else. She didn't want to see the truth, having been through this with her own mother. She prayed that she was wrong, but when he crashed the car and their doctor gave them the Alzheimer's diagnosis, and then told them that he could no longer drive…she'd felt as though someone had ripped the floor out from under her. She stopped accepting invitations from friends—always a private person, she didn't want others to pity her or know their business. She'd even tried to hide his illness from their two daughters, but as his dementia progressed to where Jim couldn't remember the names of their grandchildren, that was no longer possible. Every conversation with her daughters now left her uncomfortable and frightened as they talked about, "you have to plan" or, "what if he has to go into a home?"

She'd had to take over all of Jim's responsibilities, things she'd never done, like handling the checkbook and taking care of the house. She was constantly on edge, every day sensing that something horrible was about to happen—and it often did. Last week he'd wandered from the house and she'd frantically called the police and the fire department, who finally located him at the hardware store four miles away. She longed for a good night's sleep but stayed awake in bed most nights, worrying and listening. Always a thin woman, she'd lost her appetite and fifteen pounds. She knew that she should go to a doctor, but everything seemed like too much effort—even getting dressed in the morning or putting on lipstick. Why bother?

A clinical depression is a sustained sad or unhappy mood. To meet diagnostic criteria through the *DSM-IV-TR* (the manual used by mental health professionals to diagnose mental illnesses), it must persist for at least two weeks, cause impairment in the person's ability to function, and have at least five of the following symptoms:

- **Sleep.** People who are depressed often experience unwanted changes in their sleep pattern. This will range from difficulty falling asleep and middle-of-the-night-arousals to waking up earlier and earlier. In some types of depression, instead of sleeping less, some people will stay in bed and feel constantly tired.

- **Interest.** When depressed, people lose interest in things they usually enjoy. This can progress to a total lack of pleasure referred to as "anhedonia."

- **Guilt.** Here we're talking about guilt that is excessive and out of proportion to the situation. For example, someone who always pays her taxes on time and never cheats becomes consumed by the belief that the IRS is coming after her. More typically, a depressed person will ruminate about everything wrong they've ever done. Their self-esteem is at rock bottom, and they can feel worthless. You may hear them say things like: "It's all my fault" and "I can't do anything right."

- **Energy.** Energy is usually decreased. People feel run down, drained, and tired. For some, depression has additional physical complaints that include generalized aches and an increased focus on medical concerns. This is especially true among older individuals.

- **Concentration.** People with depression may have trouble focusing. As the depression worsens, even focusing on a television show or reading a short newspaper article may become too much.

- **Appetite.** It's most common for people with depression to lose their appetite, along with quite a bit of weight. Some people, however, eat constantly and gain weight.

- **Psychomotor agitation or slowing.** This refers to how the person looks and feels. Sometimes people with depression can be markedly slowed, their speech diminished to one or two-word answers and the expression on their face flat and unchanging. Or they could be visibly anxious, worried, and jumpy—this could be called a 'hand-wringing' depression.

- **Suicide.** People who are in unbearable psychological pain often think of suicide as a way out. Expressed thoughts of suicide should always be taken seriously, as most people who kill themselves (over 90 percent) have told someone that they were thinking about it. In addition, caregivers who think of suicide should also be assessed for the presence of homicidal thinking. In the previous vignette, for example, it would be important to find out if Claire were also having thoughts of killing her husband.

What can I do to get over my depression?

It's important to know that depression is a highly treatable condition. Even though you or someone you love is suffering and feels there is no hope—there is. If you think you may be depressed, even just a little, talk with your health care provider. If the person with dementia who you care for is currently being followed at a geriatric or dementia clinic, it's possible they will have you fill out questionnaires on a regular basis to determine how stressed out or depressed you feel.

The treatment of depression can take a number of forms, and you should start to feel improvement within a few weeks. For caregivers, where the stress and burden have worsened the depression or even led to it, interventions will need to target this stress and try to lessen it. The approach to treating depression in a caregiver will likely include a number of the following:

- Evaluation by a mental health professional (psychiatrist, psychologist, APRN)
    - Use of antidepressant medication (see Chapter 8).
    - Inpatient hospitalization if the depression has progressed to where you are having serious thoughts of ending your own

life or someone else's life, or are so disabled by the depression you can no longer function.

- Counseling or therapy. This could be one-to-one, family-based or group-based. It may be especially useful to work with a counselor familiar with dementia and issues related to loss and the grieving process.
- Referral to a support group for caregivers, such as are offered through the Alzheimer's Association, www.alz.org.
- Referral to social service agencies, such as your area council on aging, and programs that can provide additional resources for the caregiver such as respite care, in-home services, and meal services.

How do I learn to accept help from others?

Some caregivers find it difficult to ask for help—even when they're horribly burdened and overwhelmed. There's often a sense that you *should* be able to manage on your own, and that if you don't you're somehow not measuring up. For others, asking for help feels like an imposition, especially if you're not able to return favors.

To start, it may be useful to look at reasons why you in fact do deserve help, and as much of it as you can get. As a caregiver for a person with dementia, you are putting in many hours of daily labor for which you are not getting paid. If it weren't for you, the burden of caring would ultimately fall to the taxpayer—it's a fact that people with dementia who don't have family or friends to care for them are far more likely to be placed in a nursing home, with the majority of the cost paid by Medicaid. The federal government has even done studies comparing the cost of in-home care to institutional placement and has concluded that your combined efforts are worth billions of dollars annually. You provide an important and valuable—even monetarily valuable—service.

Aside from the financial issues, there are all of the emotional, spiritual, and quality-of-life concerns that you help to alleviate. The majority of people with dementia would far prefer to stay in their own home as long as possible. They are also more likely to get better care in the home than in an institution. There can also be a great deal of personal meaning and satisfaction that comes from caring for a loved one when they are no longer able to care for themselves.

Finally, if being a competent caregiver is important to you—and it is—you need to keep yourself as emotionally and physically fit as possible. You will be less effective if you're feeling burnt out or your own health is impaired.

So if you find yourself not looking for help, or turning down offers of help, it's time to rethink your role and what you need to do it as well as possible. You need to remind yourself that what you're providing is important and meaningful, and asking for the resources you need to do this job is a part of it.

How do I deal with my anger?

- *"I know it's not his fault and he has a sickness," Carol said about her father, "but he won't even try. It's like if I don't watch him every minute he's either pulling down his pants or yelling at me for something that never happened. Sometimes I just feel like screaming at him to cut it out!"*
- *"I can't get over being angry," John told his doctor, "we both worked so hard and these were supposed to be our golden years! We were going to travel, and I was going to be a golf bum. Now, I can barely leave the home. We stopped having sex years ago, and she hardly even recognizes me."*

When someone close to you develops dementia, a number of normal emotional responses will occur; among these is anger. Anger is part of how we deal with bad news and loss; it's part of the natural grieving process. *How and why could this happen? I didn't sign on for this!*

The first step in getting through this is to acknowledge that how you feel is real and it is okay. There's no shame in being mad when something bad happens, especially if it's to someone you care about. And like layers of an onion, it's not a single thing that's gone wrong—it's many things wrapped together: new financial issues, changing roles, hopes for the future that are less likely to occur, etc.

Though the anger is natural, you need to get past it. Beyond a certain point, the anger serves no productive purpose. Being trapped and stuck with your anger makes it difficult to plan and regroup around the present and the future. Also, anger directed toward the person with dementia can be sensed from your facial expression or tone of voice and may worsen their behavioral problems. If trying to provide care in the bathroom or at meal time leads to shouting and outbursts, both you and the person you care for will be left feeling horrible and drained.

So here are some strategies to help you move past your anger. Be aware that this is probably not a one-time thing, so developing—and practicing—methods to calm the anger will be useful.

- Acceptance. This happens when you acknowledge that the reality is what it is, and no amount of anger, depression, or denial will change that. It doesn't mean that you have to like the situation, just that you accept it.
- Family and friends. When angry, call up a supportive friend or family member and vent. Better yet, invite them over.
- Humor. As bleak as things can sometimes appear, do you have the ability to find something about it funny? It's okay to be irreverent. Humor and laughter are truly infectious and if you

can find a way to make yourself smile or laugh, it's likely that the person you're caring for will follow along. To help, keep a stack of funny videos or comedy tapes easily accessible and joke around with the person you're caring for to see if you can get them to laugh.

- Prayer and spiritual support. If your spiritual life has been important to you, consider strengthening it through daily prayer or regular church/temple/mosque attendance.
- Mindfulness and meditation. Can you catch yourself in the moment and identify what you are feeling and thinking? Without judging, let the thoughts and emotions pass; focus on the present and changing moment. Consider taking a mindfulness, yoga, or meditation class, and make time on a daily basis to practice.
- Find a support group, and attend it. Being around others who are going through the same or similar things can be uplifting and validating.
- Shake it off. Sometimes physical activity such as exercise, even just taking a walk or working in the garden, can calm your mood. Daily exercise has been shown to have antidepressant properties in addition to its other benefits.
- Do something else. If you find yourself getting upset and angry while doing a particular task (bathing, dressing, feeding) with a person with dementia, it may be that the best thing—if you can—is to do something else and then return to the task when you're calm.

How important is having a support group?

Research shows that one of the best ways for caregivers to battle their stress is to become educated about dementia and learn strategies to deal with all of the related issues that pop up. For many people, the best place to get this information is from others who have gone through it, or are currently caring for someone with dementia. Some support groups—such as the four-session family education group offered by the Alzheimer's Association—are specifically geared toward giving caregivers and families information and education.

In addition to information—such as which is the best adult day care in town, which elder law attorneys seem to really know their stuff, and which nursing home has the most sensitive staff— support groups provide a place for caregivers to come together for encouragement and camaraderie. There's also a certain reality that people find in support groups, which may be easier to relate to than a health care professional offering advice. For instance, if someone else has a loved one for whom showering was a big issue, you may be able to take strategies they have found helpful and use them in your own situation.

Over time, support groups that stick together develop strong bonds among the members, which can extend to friendships and social networks that go outside the boundaries of the weekly or monthly group setting.

Where do I find a support group?

The largest resource for Alzheimer's support groups is through the Alzheimer's Association. For locations and schedules of groups near you, they can be contacted at their twenty-four-hour help line— 800–356–5502—or on the Internet at www.alz.org/ct/in_my_community_support.asp.

The Alzheimer's Association also hosts several chat rooms and message boards that are geared toward specific groups or topics, such as a group for people with Alzheimer's, groups for caregivers, and groups for providers. The direct link for this is http://www. alz.org/

living_with_alzheimers_message_boards_lwa.asp. Finally, there may be support groups in your local area run through religious organizations, senior centers, hospitals, or other institutions. Ask around and attend different meetings to find out where you feel the most comfortable and where you get the most help.

What is respite care?

Respite care is anything that provides a break from round-the-clock caregiving duties. Respite care can be provided in the home—such as with an aide or therapist—or can be hours, days, or up to a couple of weeks out of the home in a skilled nursing facility. Adult day care programs (see Chapter 7) are a form of respite. Some convalescent centers offer extended respite and some agencies, such as the Alzheimer's Association and your state's branch of the Administration on Aging (AOA), can occasionally assist families in paying for brief respite admissions.

Respite programs can be a real lifesaver to help rejuvenate care-givers who are feeling burdened and need a break. For caregivers who have been unable to take a vacation or visit family out-of-state for an important event, finding a respite program may be what you need to recharge your emotional batteries.

How can I maintain a social life if my husband has dementia?

"Ever since Dave was diagnosed with Alzheimer's we stopped going out. I get too nervous that he'll wander off or do something that will embar-rass us in front of our friends."

Caregivers, especially those looking after an ill spouse or signifi-cant other, are often reluctant to keep up with their prior social activities—friends, clubs, family gatherings, religious services, and so forth. The reasons for this are varied and may be a combination of practical and emotional factors—lack of someone to look after the person with dementia when you're out of the house, embarrassment over having to explain why your spouse is no longer with you, feeling too tired or stressed to relax in a social situation, etc. Or for some couples, everything they did was done together. Now that one of the partners is no longer able to participate in usual social activities, the well spouse is in unfamiliar territory and may not feel comfortable going out on their own.

The big problem with having your social life shrink is that you lose important emotional supports and healthy outlets that give you pleasure and help you recharge your batteries. So, what to do? First, you need to give yourself permission to have a social life. It's important and will help you maintain your overall sense of well-being, and if you're not healthy, you can't properly care for anyone else. Next, you need to decide whether to include the person with dementia in the activity. If so, it will be a matter of thinking through the event to decrease the chances of there being a problem. This might include enlisting the help of one or two other friends or family members, to share in any oversight that might be needed. If it doesn't make sense—for whatever reason—to bring the person with dementia, then it's a matter of getting the right level of in-home care in place.

And if going out has become too difficult, or can only be done on rare occasions, find ways of bringing your friends and family to you. This can be as simple as regular phone calls, visits, and small get-togethers.

I don't want everyone to know that John has Alzheimer's; is this wrong?

"My wife has always been a very private person. She just wouldn't want everyone knowing her business."

There are valid reasons why people decide to disclose, or not disclose, their loved one's Alzheimer's or dementia. There is no one right answer, and often people only disclose the diagnosis to close friends and family. If you decide not to talk about the illness, it may be important to look at the reasons behind this decision. Is it a desire to maintain someone's privacy? Or does the diagnosis feel like a shameful secret that must be kept quiet? While this might seem far-fetched, this attitude toward illnesses in general runs strong in our culture. It wasn't that long ago that even mentioning the word "cancer" was considered a type of taboo.

While there is nothing wrong with keeping the information private, there is a real positive side to being able to freely talk about the illness. It helps inform people about Alzheimer's and dementia, and works to decrease the stigma by putting a human face on the disorder. More importantly, because dementia is so widespread and has affected most families at one time or another, a common response is, "I know exactly what you're going through; I looked after my father for the last four years of his life." By opening up, you might be surprised how many people will share their stories and support.

Chapter 17

IF YOU'VE BEEN DIAGNOSED

- How do I get on with my life after I've been diagnosed with Alzheimer's?
- I feel like my children are running my life—how do I get them to back off?
- Should I tell my friends that I've been diagnosed with an early dementia?
- How do I handle my children fighting over my care?
- What can I do to prevent going into a nursing home?
- Is it okay to start a new relationship if I know I have a dementia?
- Are there support groups for me?

How do I get on with my life after I've been diagnosed with Alzheimer's?

"For some time now, I've known my memory is slipping. My wife kept telling me it was nothing. I can see that she's almost more afraid than I am. There's so much that I still want to do. Is this the end of all of that, of all our dreams?"

Awareness of dementia and Alzheimer's is highest in the early stages, as can be depression and a profound sense of loss. With work and support, getting through this tough time can be done with grace and humor; however, if things have progressed to a point where you are sad all the time, have no sense of a future, and derive little to no pleasure out of life, you may have a clinical depression, which requires treatment (see questions on depression in Chapter 9). It's important to remember that depression—even the depression that can come with dementia—is a treatable condition.

There are a number of things that can help you deal with the diagnosis and get to a general sense of acceptance. First off, your life is not over, and you may well have a number of years where you can still do quite a bit. It's a fact that everybody dies. For you, what's different is that you've been given a diagnosis that forces you to look at your own mortality. In general, we don't like to do this—but there can be something of a silver lining. The diagnosis can be a wake-up call and an opportunity to get your affairs—emotional, relationship, spiritual, and financial—into order. If you've not drawn up a will and advance directives (see Chapter 13), it's important to not procrastinate and get all of that taken care of. If there is a trip or some other big activity you've been putting off, maybe now is the time.

Find those things and people that have given you support at other times in your life, be they family, friends, religious groups, or even favorite activities. Chances are good that they will help now. While there is often an impulse to withdraw from people when we are emotionally hurt or physically ill, this can be a time to reinvest in important relationships. Let people know that you're okay and that you're planning to get through this. Let them know what your wishes are for the future and by all means let the people you care about know how you feel. If you're able to embrace a positive attitude, those around you will feel comfortable following your lead.

For some, adopting a "carpe diem" ("seize the day") approach can be helpful. Yes, you've been given a diagnosis that will impair your abilities at some time in the future—but if today is a good day, make the best of it.

I feel like my children are running my life—how do I get them to back off?

"I know my daughter Megan means well. But she's constantly telling me what to do and rearranges all of my things so I can't find anything. I like my cupboards set up the way they are and don't want her messing around in them. And I like to leave my food on the counter so I can see what I have and don't have to bend down to get to everything."

Roles between parents and children often get turned around when a parent becomes ill or develops Alzheimer's. As a result, two major tensions develop—you have the child or caregiver who wants to keep their parent or loved one safe, and you have the person with dementia, who may view all of this "helpfulness" as an intrusion and bossiness. The trick is to find the middle ground that provides a degree of safety and allows the person with dementia to not feel that they are being treated like a child. This approach gets even more challenging when we factor in the progressive nature of most dementias—this middle ground may be totally different six months later.

For the caregiver, the approach needs to be one of 'do no more than the person needs done.' If someone is still caring for their own home, there's no need to step in, even if it's not as spick-and-span as you might want. If it's not unhealthy or filthy, and your cleaning assistance is not requested or desired, let things go. When you must step in for safety or other reasons, try to do so in a way that helps preserve the person's dignity and sense of autonomy. Avoid making ultimatums, such as "you must do this" and look for ways you can offer choices: "Where would you like me to put this?"

For the person with dementia, it will involve being as active and on top of things as possible. Clearly this is more for someone with an early dementia, but incorporating routines—such as pill boxes, written schedules, and to-do lists—and sticking to them will help support your independence, and let others see you are doing well enough to be independent. It's important to remember that your family's intrusiveness is probably generated by their concern for you. To help make them feel more comfortable, there are a number of things you can do that will help reassure them that you're okay.

- Consider installing a personal emergency alarm in your home, including a button you can wear around your neck should you have a fall or require emergency medical assistance. These can quite literally be a life saver.
- Frequent—even daily—check-in phone calls with family can let them know you're doing okay.
- Schedule regular activities with family or concerned care-givers—such as shopping trips, meals, religious activities, or recreational activities.

Should I tell my friends that I've been diagnosed with an early dementia?

While it's probably not important to let casual friends know about your diagnosis, you may want to broach the topic with people you are close to. It doesn't need to be scary and filled with medical details; it could be as simple as, "I've been having problems with my memory, and the doctors tell me it's going to get worse as time goes on."

People will normally respond by asking one or two follow-up questions, or they might offer some information from their own life: *"Like Alzheimer's? My aunt had that."* If your friends see that you're handling the diagnosis well, their response will generally match yours. In disclosing your diagnosis there is the risk that someone may be frightened by the information and pull away from you. However, if they are indeed a good friend, letting them into your confidence will ease any burden you feel from keeping your diagnosis a secret and it will offer your friend the opportunity to be there for you.

How do I handle my children fighting over my care?

In addition to writing down your advance directives and giving copies to key people in your life, as discussed in Chapter 13, it's important to maintain a good flow of dialogue with concerned family members. If you have particular likes and dislikes regarding treatment, you need to make these known. In the absence of your input, it's common for family members—your children, especially— to disagree over what they believe you'd want or what should be done. This can create volatile situations in emergency rooms and hospitals: one child may say, "do everything possible," another says "Dad wouldn't want that," and a third is put in the position of trying to keep the peace.

While many people don't want to talk about what to do should they become ill, these frank discussions with your children, spouse/partner, and other important people in your life can prove invaluable in a time of need. By letting them know what you want, you relieve them of making the decision and the resulting intense feelings of guilt, anger, and confusion.

What can I do to prevent going into a nursing home?

The majority of people with dementia would prefer to stay in their own homes. Most caregivers would like this as well. Home is where we feel comfortable, and if you're already having problems with memory and confusion, a new and unfamiliar setting can make things worse. Figuring out how you can remain in your own home starts with an assessment of your particular situation. The assessment involves a few basic questions:

- Is the home safe?
- Are you getting your basic needs met (food, clothing, shelter, personal hygiene, medical care)?
- Can you afford to maintain the home?

Each of these questions will involve specific things that need to be done, and because dementias change over time, you'll need backup plans—what do you need now, and what might you need in the future? Things you should do may include:

- Be clear with family members and/or friends and loved ones that your goal is to remain in your own home.
- Have advance directives that allow for various "what if?" situations so that whoever will be making decisions for you can do what needs to be done to keep you in your own home.
- Arrange your finances so that paying for home maintenance, in-home care, and any other necessary services is set up well in advance.

Is it okay to start a new relationship if I know I have a dementia?

Enjoying every day and living life to the fullest includes maintaining important friendships and relationships and allowing for the possibility of new ones. If you're someone who has always enjoyed getting involved in group trips and activities, there's little reason to stop, especially in the early stages of a dementia. It would be prudent to buddy up with someone, so that should you become disoriented in a new surrounding—such as on a museum trip or other activity—they can be in charge of getting you both back to the bus on time.

Staying involved in social activities, including religious, community, and family events, will help keep you healthy and emotionally well. And if you find yourself making a connection with a new person, as in every other stage of life, this is a gift that can be enjoyed.

Are there support groups for me?

While not as numerous as the support groups for family members and caregivers, there are support groups for people with dementia. There are also support groups for couples in which one partner has a dementia and the other does not. The best source of information about where these groups are, when they meet, etc., will be through your local Alzheimer's Association and can be located through their website, www.alz.org. The site also has chat groups for people with dementia.

Chapter 18

THE FAMILY

- What is the sandwich generation?
- How do I make time for both my children and my mother with Alzheimer's?
- How do I explain an elder relative's dementia to our children?
- Should I include my grandmother with dementia in family events?
- How do I get my brothers and sisters to help take care of Dad?
- What do I do if my siblings won't help out?
- What do I do if no one in the family agrees with me that Mom is no longer safe in her home?

What is the sandwich generation?

- *"There is absolutely no way I can be with Mom all the time. Who's going to get Janice to cheerleading and Tommy to soccer? And I work...this just isn't realistic. There's no way I can do all of this."*

- *"I'm a single dad and I wish my brothers and sister would lay off about my 'doing my share' for Dad. I don't have the time, and frankly, they do. It's not like I don't love him, it's just he can't be my top priority right now when I have two small children of my own, especially when my sister doesn't have kids and my brothers live much closer."*

The sandwich generation describes men and women who are simultaneously raising children and caring for parents with disabilities such as Alzheimer's. In this double-caregiver role, people are faced with having to juggle and balance the needs and wants of different family members—children, spouse/significant other, and parents.

This group often experiences difficult challenges and choices, not least of which is financial. With many single-income or single-parent families, it's easy to see how caring for Mom, the kids, and keeping a job to pay the bills could become an overwhelming burden.

How do I make time for both my children and my mother with Alzheimer's?

When you are a parent and a caregiver at the same time, it can feel like you are being stretched beyond what is manageable. Even if the person you're caring for is in a home or institution, there are regular demands on your time and emotions. Finding ways to strike a balance with the needs of your children, your husband/ wife/significant other, and job will involve choices. This is not a question with simple answers; what works for you and your situation will be different from what works for someone else. There are many factors that need to be considered here:

- What is the situation of the person with dementia? How much care do they need? Where are they living—in their own home? With you? In an institution? Are there others to help with the caregiver responsibilities? What finances have been put in place, or are available, for this person's care?
- The ages and special needs of your children. Are you a single parent? Are there others you can rely on to help with caring for your children?
- Your work situation
- Your finances
- Your own health and that of others in your family

Those may be the most concrete concerns, but there are quite a few other things you want to take into consideration: location, set-up of the home, availability of transportation, other community supports and resources, not to mention hard-to-measure things like your disposition, the natures of your children, and the overall emotional and behavioral condition of the person with dementia. You need to know if you'll be able to strategize ways to free up or arrange your time so that you can be there for your children and the person requiring care.

This overview of your situation is a complex equation with many variables. It's worth spending some time thinking through it to see where you may have some opportunity to rearrange and organize your time and resources. The following represent a few areas where you may be able to make some changes. This is not an exhaustive list, and the solutions caregivers come up with—because there are so many factors involved—are often very creative and completely unique.

- Establish and stick to regular family routines that your children can depend on as being "together time"—meals, after supper homework or TV time, weekend activities together.
- As appropriate, include your children in activities with the person with dementia.
- Is respite care an option for you (see Chapter 16)? Are there respite grants available in your community for adult day care or in-home assistance?
- Are you or the person with dementia able to pay for day care or other paid caregiving assistance out-of-pocket? Is there long-term insurance that will help cover this cost?
- Are there other family members or friends who can help out with the caregiving responsibilities? If so, get a regular commitment.
- Are you spending too much time traveling between locations—your home, work, children's activities, errands, and the location of the person with dementia? Is there some change you could make here that would cut out hours of travel time, like moving the person with dementia closer, arranging a carpool for your kids, automating some of your errands, etc.?
- Are there things you can do with your work/job schedule that might make a positive change at home? Obviously, this is a wide-open suggestion. Many caregivers find they need to cut back at work, while others with better earning potential may shift more of their income to purchasing assistance in the home—nannies, au pairs, paid caregivers for the person with dementia.
- Are there other time-consuming activities, errands, or chores you currently do that could be given to someone else, like laundry, housekeeping, yard work, etc.?

How do I explain an elder relative's dementia to our children?

- *"Why does Grandma keep telling the same story over and over? Doesn't she know I've heard it like a million times?"*
- *"Daddy just called me Bobby; doesn't he know I'm his son and not his brother?"*
- *"Grandpa won't stop crying. What's wrong with him?"*
- *"Mom keeps trying to get into my room at night. She's really freaking me out."*

Children and teens, depending on their age and level of maturity, intelligence, etc., will experience the behavior of family members with dementia in a variety of ways. Much will also depend on the person's stage of dementia and whatever behaviors they're exhibiting.

The best approach is to talk to your children in a clear and simple fashion. With younger children you'll want to let them know that the person is ill and they can no longer remember things the way they used to. It's also important to let them know that if they ever are frightened or scared by anything the person with dementia does or says, they should immediately come to you or another adult.

Helping children feel comfortable with a person who has dementia might include teaching them to roll with some of the things the person with dementia may say. It's also important to show them that they can still share time with the person who has dementia, do activities together, laugh, and enjoy their company.

- *"Dear, even if you tell Grandma thirty times that she's living in our house and not hers, she won't remember. So if it gets her upset, just stop doing it."*
- *"Mom, I had such a good time working in the garden with Grandpa today!"*

With your help, guidance, and example your children can learn important lessons about caring for others, and how illness is a part of life and not something to hide away. Allowing children to participate in caring for someone will also help them develop compassion, empathy, and patience.

Should I include my grandmother with dementia in family events?

Including family members with dementia in important events—weddings, holidays, birthday parties, etc.—will depend on how the person is doing, whether or not they will be able to tolerate the stimulation of the event, and if they will actually derive pleasure from being there. It's also important to consider whether *you* can derive pleasure from the event with them there.

In the earlier stages of dementia, you may have few concerns about including the person. If it's going to be in a strange setting, or they are prone to wandering, you will want someone to be given the task of keeping an eye on them. In moderate and advanced dementia the decision to include the person will need to take into account how well they tolerate unfamiliar settings, and whether or not they are prone to behavioral outbursts. If you believe the person will be able to handle the event it would be wise to have either a family member, or paid caregiver, be with them and assist them as needed—finding the bathroom, help with the meal. It might also be helpful to limit the person's time at the event and to have an emergency exit plan if a problem occurs.

How do I get my brothers and sisters to help take care of Dad?

If you are the primary caregiver for a parent or parents with dementia, getting help from other relatives, especially your brothers and sisters, may become a significant issue. In general, what you want is help with the overall burden of being a caregiver. This assistance can come in three forms: emotional, financial, and help in freeing up some of your time. The best way to go about this is to be direct and just ask. It's probably best to do this early on, even if you're someone who has always struggled with asking others for help. What's not a good idea is letting resentment bottle up and then blasting family members with a laundry list of complaints you've accumulated over the last three years. Be clear with what you need:

- *"It's costing about $350 a week for Dad's adult day care; how much can you kick in?"*
- *"Even with her insurance Mom's meds are over $500 a month; can you go half?"*
- *"If I don't get some time away from Mom she's going to drive me bonkers. I need you to take her on the weekends; can you do that?"*
- *"I just need to vent. She got all upset and was convinced I'd stolen her underwear and sold it."*

What do I do if my siblings won't help out?

The sad reality is that, when we need help, even our family might not always be there for us. When you're the primary caregiver and your adult brothers and sisters aren't shouldering what you believe is their fair share, this has the potential to be a whole new source of stress. Probably the best way to handle this is to break it down into a few fairly simple steps.

1. Identify the reason(s) why someone is not able or willing to help out.
   a. They live too far away.
   b. They're struggling financially.

c. They have not yet accepted that their parent has a dementia, or that it is as serious as it is.

d. They disagree with how you are handling the caregiver role.

2. Negotiate and try to identify specific ways in which they might be able to help.

a. *"I know that money's tight, what could you come up with? Anything will help right now."*

b. *"You know what I'd like more than money? If you could take Mom shopping, to the beauty parlor, and to a couple of her doctor's appointments, that would be great."*

c. *"I didn't realize you still thought she was doing better. I've got a copy of her evaluation and the psychological testing, I'll make you a copy."*

3. If negotiation is not successful, or they are flat-out unwilling to pitch in, for your own well-being you may have to accept this, not necessarily like it, and move on. It doesn't mean that you don't deserve the emotional, financial, and other support, just that you will have to look elsewhere, such as friends, support groups, and financial assistance and programs that may be available through your area agency on aging, local Alzheimer's Association, church, senior center, etc.

What do I do if no one in the family agrees with me that Mom is no longer safe in her home?

When you start discussing family interactions, things are likely to get complicated. Old grudges and rivalries emerge, and conflicts that we thought we left behind in childhood—*"Mom always liked you best"*—come back strong. As a result, it's common that close relatives will not always be in agreement about important treatment and care decisions that need to be made.

This is one of the reasons why having advance planning and advance directives are so important. In the best of all situations, the person with dementia, when they were still well enough, spelled out their likes and dislikes. This can go a long way toward decreasing arguments later on where people are trying to guess what their loved one would have wanted. Clearly, even the best and most thoughtful advance planning can't foresee every possibility, but if the person with dementia has appointed a health care decision-maker or durable power of attorney, this person has the ultimate responsibility for making decisions in the person's best interest. Similarly if a court has appointed a guardian or conservator, it is that person's obligation to make the decisions.

In the absence of this kind of planning, it may be useful to step back from the problem and try to look at it from a distance. In the case of someone's safety in their own home and a family disagreement over what to do, the first step may be to bring in objective outsiders and get their assessment and recommendations. Depending on the stage of dementia and how serious the danger is, this may or may not be a realistic approach—if the person with dementia needs help immediately, that takes precedence.

Things that might help you convince your family that the person with dementia needs help include:

- Get a thorough dementia evaluation (see Chapter 4) and ask them to make specific recommendations about in-home safety.
  - Involve concerned others in this evaluation and keep them up-to-date on the results.
  - Make sure involved family get copies of the official reports, including the specific recommendations.
- Consult an attorney who specializes in elder law (See Chapter 14).

- ◆ Is the person still able to handle their own affairs?
- ◆ Are they able to spell out what they'd like for advance directives?
- ◆ Do they need a guardian or conservator appointed by the court?
- If you are the primary caregiver, offer opportunities for concerned others to share in this responsibility. It may be that by giving them more firsthand opportunity to observe the situation, they will be able to see exactly what you are concerned about.

Chapter 19

HOPE FOR THE FUTURE

- Is there a cure in sight for Alzheimer's disease?
- What is immunotherapy?
- Are there new tests coming that can tell if someone is going to get Alzheimer's?
- How can I help support the fight for a cure?
- How does someone become part of a research project or drug study?
- How can someone with dementia give consent to be in a clinical trial or study?
- Are there new programs being developed that will help families and caregivers?

Is there a cure in sight for Alzheimer's disease?

This is an exciting time in the development of Alzheimer's and dementia research. The understanding of these illnesses has progressed dramatically with the development of new brain-imaging techniques and other new and improved technologies. Even more encouraging are the experimental therapies being developed and tested that may prevent and possibly even reverse some of the brain damage seen in Alzheimer's and other dementias.

It is a realistic hope that in the next five to ten years we will see new treatments that will substantially improve the course of Alzheimer's, especially for those who catch it in its earliest stages. So while a cure is not yet around the corner, the advances being made now may be the groundwork needed for a definitive cure to be found.

What is immunotherapy?

One of the most promising areas of Alzheimer's research is immunotherapy, and human studies are currently underway. This is an approach that targets the actual lesions (amyloid plaques) seen in the brains of people with Alzheimer's. In brief, various proteins are believed to be involved in the cell death associated with Alzheimer's. The protein that is most implicated is beta-amyloid (β-amyloid).

Immunotherapy involves introducing another protein, called an immunoglobulin, that attaches to the amyloid and removes it from the brain and from the body. This is the same principle used when getting immunized against a particular disease, such as hepatitis or the mumps. The immunoglobulin recognizes its target, attaches to it in a lock-and-key fashion, and this combination is then able to be broken down and removed from the body.

Immunotherapy for dementia was first studied in mice that were genetically altered to have Alzheimer's disease. The results published in 1999 were quite promising—reduction in amyloid plaques and improved functioning in the mice. However, the second human study that followed needed to be discontinued because the substance was too toxic in approximately 6 percent of those receiving it. Studies looking at those who had undergone the treatment did show slowing of the disease, and the autopsy of one patient who died twenty months after the treatment showed a reduction in the number of amyloid plaques in her brain.

Less toxic immunotherapy compounds have since been developed and are currently undergoing large-scale human investigations that will hopefully lead to useful therapies in the next five to ten years.

Are there new tests coming that can tell if someone is going to get Alzheimer's?

While there are currently no blood tests available that can reliably tell whether or not someone has Alzheimer's or will develop it, there are some promising new developments. New diagnostic tests being developed include ones that look at subtle differences between proteins found in the blood of people with Alzheimer's and those who don't have it; one promising, but very preliminary, study underway has been able to identify the blood of people with Alzheimer's disease with 90 percent accuracy. In this same study they were also able to identify those people with mild cognitive impairment who later developed the full-blown disease with 80 percent accuracy.

How can I help support the fight for a cure?

Research is the key to finding better treatments for Alzheimer's and other dementias. Finding ways that you can support this research—either financially or by participating in a study—are the major ways you can help. Contact the Alzheimer's Association (www.alz.org) to find out the best ways you can help.

How does someone become part of a research project or drug study?

There is a tremendous amount of research currently going on in the field of dementia, and Alzheimer's in particular. Some studies focus on clinical trials of new medications, some look at imaging techniques to better identify and diagnose, while others look at strategies to help caregivers. Research into Alzheimer's is funded through various sources, which include governmental agencies such as the National Institute of Health (NIH), not-for-profit organizations like the Alzheimer's Association, and pharmaceutical companies looking to evaluate the effectiveness of medications.

Around the country there are more than thirty research centers funded by the U.S. National Institutes of Health's National Institute on Aging. Each of these centers participates in a range of research activities for which they need test subjects. If you think you might want to become involved in a research project, contact the center closest to you for information about current studies or search their website for current clinical trials at http://www.nia.nih.gov/ Alzheimers/ResearchInformation/ClinicalTrials. In addition, your state's Alzheimer's Association may be aware of studies currently looking for test subjects—www.alzheimer's.org.

Arizona Alzheimer's Center	Boston University
Arizona Alzheimer's Disease Consortium (ADC)	Bedford VA Medical Center
Banner Alzheimer's Institute	GRECC Program (182B)
901 E Willetta St.	200 Springs Road
Phoenix, AZ 85006	Bedford, MA 01730
Tel: 602–239–6999	Tel: 781–687–2632
Fax: 602–239–6253	Fax: 781–687–3515
Website: http://alzheimers.sbs.arizona.edu/	Website: http://www.bu.edu/alzresearch/

Case Western Reserve University [INACTIVE] Case Western Reserve University 2109 Adelbert Road, Rm. E653 Cleveland, OH 44106 Tel: 216–368–6101 Fax: 216–368–3079 Website: http://www.memoryandagingcenter.org	**Columbia University** Columbia University, Department of Pathology 630 W 168th St., P&S 15–402 New York, NY 10032 Tel: 212–305–3300 Fax: 212–305–5498 Website: http://www.alzheimercenter.org
Duke University Medical Center Duke University Medical Center Bryan ADRC 2200 W Main St., Suite A-200 Durham, NC 27705 Tel: 919–668–0820 Fax: 919–668–0828 Website: http://adrc.mc.duke.edu	**Emory University** Emory University, Neurology Department 101 Woodruff Circle #6000 Atlanta, GA 30322 Tel: 404–727–7220 Fax: 404–727–3999 Website: http://www.med.Emory.edu/ADRC
Florida Alzheimer's Center Byrd Alzheimer's Institute 15310 Amberly Dr., Suite 320 Tampa, FL 33647 Tel: 813–866–1600 Fax: 813–866–1601 Website: http://www.byrdinstitute.org	**Indiana University School of Medicine** Indiana University School of Medicine Department of Pathology & Lab Medicine 635 Barnhill Dr., MS A138 Indianapolis, IN 46202 Tel: 317–274–7818 Fax: 317–274–4882 Website: http://iadc.iupui.edu
Johns Hopkins University School of Medicine Johns Hopkins University School of Medicine 720 Rutland Avenue, 558 Ross Baltimore, MD 21205–2196 Tel: 410–502–5169 Fax: 410–955–9777 Website: http://www.alzresearch.org	**Massachusetts General Hospital** Massachusetts General Hospital CNY 114, Room 2009 Charlestown, MA 02129 Tel: 617–726–2299 Fax: 617–724–1480 Website: http://www.madrc.org

Mayo Clinic Mayo Clinic, Department of Neurology 200 First St. SW Rochester, MN 55905 Tel: 507–538–0487 Fax: 507–538–6012 Website: http://mayoresearch.mayo.edu/may o/research/alzheimers_center	**Mount Sinai School of Medicine** Mount Sinai School of Medicine Department of Psychiatry One Gustave Levy Place, Box 1230 New York, NY 10029 Tel: 718–741–4228 Fax: 718–562–9120 Website: http://www.mssm.edu/psychiatry/adrc/
New York University New York University, ADRC, Millhauser Labs 560 First Avenue New York, NY 10016 Tel: 212–263–5703 Fax: 212–263–6991 Website: http://aging.med.nyu.edu/programs /alzheimers/	**Northwestern University** Northwestern University Medical School 675 N St. Clair, Galter 20–100 Chicago, IL 60611 Tel: 312–908–9339 Fax: 312–908–8789 Website: http://www.brain.northwestern.edu
Oregon Health and Science University Oregon Health & Science University Aging & Alzheimer Disease Center CR131 3181 SW Sam Jackson Park Road Portland, OR 97239–3098 Tel: 503–494–6976 Fax: 503–494–7499 Website: http://www.ohsu.edu/som-alzheimers/oadc_page.html	**Rush University Medical Center** Rush University Medical Center Armour Academic Center 600 S Paulina St., Suite 1028 Chicago, IL 60612 Tel: 312–942–2362 Fax: 312–563–4605 Website: http://www.rush.edu/rumc/page-R12388.html

Stanford University [INACTIVE]	University of Alabama, Birmingham
Stanford University Department of Psychiatry, 5550 401 Quarry Road, C305 Palo Alto, CA 94305–5717 Tel: 650–852–3287 Fax: 650–852–3297 Website: http://alzheimer.stanford.edu	University of Alabama at Birmingham Sparks Research Center 1720 7th Ave. S, Suite 650K Birmingham, Alabama 35233–7340 Tel: 205–934–2334 Fax: 205–975–3094 Website: http://main.uab.edu/show.asp?durki=11627
University of Arkansas [INACTIVE]	**University of California, Davis**
University of Arkansas for Medical Sciences Department of Geriatrics 4301 W Markham, Slot 808 Little Rock, Arkansas 72205–7199 Tel: 501–526–5750 Fax: 501–526–5760 Website: http://alzheimer.uams.edu	University of California Davis Medical Center 4860 Y Street, Suite 3700 Sacramento, CA 95817 Tel: 916–734–8413 Fax: 916–734–6525 Website: http://alzheimer.ucdavis.edu/
University of California, Irvine	**University of California, Los Angeles**
University of California, Irvine Gillespie NRF, Rm. 1113 Irvine, CA 92697–4540 Tel: 949–824–5847 Fax: 949–824–2071 Website: http://www.alz.uci.edu/	University of California, Los Angeles 10911 Weyburn Ave., Suite 200 Los Angeles, CA 90095–7226 Tel: 310–794–3665 Fax: 310–794–3148 Website: http://www.adc.ucla.edu
University of California, San Diego	**University of California, San Francisco**
UCSD School of Medicine 9500 Gilman Drive (0624) La Jolla, CA 92093–0624 Tel: 858–534–8585 Fax: 858–534–2985 Website: http://adrc.ucsd.edu/	University of California, San Francisco Box 1207 350 Parnassus Ave, #706 San Francisco, CA 94143–1207 Tel: 415–476–6242 Fax: 415–476–4800 Website: http://www.memory.ucsf.edu/

University of Kentucky	University of Michigan
University of Kentucky 101 Sanders-Brown Center on Aging 800 S Limestone St. Lexington, KY 40536–0230 Tel: 859–323–6040 Fax: 859–323–2866 Website: http://www.mc.uky.edu/coa/ADRC/adrc.htm	University of Michigan Department of Neurology 300 N Ingalls 3D15 Ann Arbor, MI 48109–0489 Tel: 734–936–1808 Fax: 734–763–1752 Website: http://www.med.umich.edu/alzheimers/
University of Pennsylvania	**University of Pittsburgh**
University of Pennsylvania 3rd Floor Maloney Building 3600 Spruce Street Philadelphia PA 19104–4283 Tel: 215–662–4708 Fax: 215–349–5909 Website: http://www.uphs.upenn.edu/ADC/	University of Pittsburgh Department of Neurology 3471 Fifth Avenue, Suite 811 Pittsburgh, PA 15213 Tel: 412–692–4622 Fax: 412–692–4526 Website: http://www.adrc.pitt.edu
University of Texas Southwestern	**University of Washington**
University of Texas Southwestern Medical Center 5323 Harry Hines Boulevard Dallas TX 75390–9036 Tel: 214–648–3239 Fax: 214–648–6824 Website: http://www.utsouthwestern.edu/alz heimers/research	VA Puget Sound Health Care System Mental Health Services, S-116 1660 S Columbian Way Seattle, WA 98108 Tel: 206–768–5375 Fax: 206–764–2573 Website: http://depts.washington.edu/adrcweb/
Washington University School of Medicine	
Washington University School of Medicine Department of Neurology Campus Box 8111, 4488 Forest Park Avenue, Suite 130 St Louis, MO 63108–2293 Tel: 314–286–2881, Fax: 314–286–2763 Website: http://alzheimer.wustl.edu/	

How can someone with dementia give consent to be in a clinical trial or study?

- *"I just saw an announcement for a new drug trial. They're looking for human subjects who have moderate dementia. I'd love to get my dad signed up; how do I do this?"*
- *"It would mean a lot to me if I could contribute to the fight against Alzheimer's. I realize that down the road I might not be able to give permission to be a research subject; is there any way I can give permission now for studies that might come up in the future?"*

Whenever human subjects are used in research, various ethical issues need to be addressed. To ensure that this happens, all research with human subjects is conducted under the supervision of institutional review boards (IRBs) that ensure that people's rights, dignity, and best interest are preserved.

For people with Alzheimer's and dementia, one of the big questions that needs to be answered is if the person is able to give informed consent to participate in a particular study. Several factors will help determine whether or not a person with dementia can enroll, or be enrolled, in a research protocol such as a trial of a new medication.

- How risky is the study? For a study with low or no risk of harm, a person with dementia—or their decision-maker/ proxy/power of attorney—should be able to enroll without difficulty. As potential risks increase, a greater deal of scrutiny will go into whether or not the person or their proxy is able to give adequate consent for the study. An example of a low-risk study might include interviews with caregivers and people with dementia about their perceived level of stress. A high-risk study could be a trial of a brand new medication, where the potential side effects or risk of adverse reactions are not fully known.

- Potential benefit. What is the potential gain this person can get out of the study? If the chance for clinical improvement is great, that gets weighed into the overall decision.
- Is the person still competent to make their own decisions? Do they understand the risks and benefits of the study? If the person has had a judge appoint a conservator or guardian, any decision to enroll in a study will need to include that person. If no conservator/guardian has been appointed and no advance directives have been completed, a family member or primary caregiver may be able to help.
- Did the person make a specific advance directive around research when they were still able to do so? The Alzheimer's Association recommends that if a person with Alzheimer's would like to be included in research, they make a specific advance directive around the types of studies in which they'd want to participate.
- Does the person with dementia have a health care decision-maker or proxy who can look out for their best interest? In the absence of a formal proxy, a family member or primary care-giver may be able to help with giving consent for certain studies.

Are there new programs being developed that will help families and caregivers?

At present there are a number of new programs being developed, funded, and implemented that will allow people with dementia and their caregivers to have greater choice, especially as it relates to keeping people in their own homes as long as possible. These programs are attempting to address the strong desire by most Americans to be cared for in their home instead of in an extended-care facility. The challenge here has been that many people cannot afford the level of in-home and community-based care needed by a person with moderate to severe dementia. As a result, when the person's needs have exceeded what they can afford or their caregivers can provide, the person must go into a nursing home, exhaust their financial resources, and then get placed on Medicaid, which covers the cost of ongoing nursing home care.

One such program that has been funded by the Department of Health and Human Services/Centers for Medicare and Medicaid Services is called "Money Follows the Person," which allows for more flexible funding of Medicaid services. This program is now in its second phase, with a five-year project (January 1, 2007, to September 30, 2011) being studied in states that applied and were awarded this grant. They're looking at ways that long-term care can be shifted from institutions such as nursing homes and hospitals, and back into less-restrictive settings such as the person's own home, a caregiver's home, or other more normal surroundings. States awarded these grants have been tasked with developing creative ways to promote personal choice, especially as it relates to keeping people out of institutional settings while still getting the level of care and support they need.

Though this program is still in its early stages, two important findings are clear. First, by shifting Medicaid funds into the community and the home, people are able to have greater choice about where they live and are cared for. And second, there appears to be a substantial cost-saving in shifting care from the nursing home back into the person's own home. It is quite possible that as this project progresses, it will be expanded so that people with dementia and their caregivers in the coming years will have greater choice and more available resources, both for in-home and for community-based services.

Appendix A

CHAPTER-BY-CHAPTER REFERENCES

Chapter 1: What Are Alzheimer's and Dementia?

Berchtold, N.C., and C. W. Cotman. Evolution in the conceptualization of dementia and Alzheimer's disease: Greco-Roman period to the 1960s. *Neurobiology of Aging* 19 (3): 173–189.

Centers for Disease Control. Characteristics and health of caregivers and care recipients—North Carolina, 2005. *Morbidity and Mortality Weekly* 56 (21): 529–532.

Hebert, L., P. Scherr, J. Bienias, D. Bennett, and D. Evans. Alzheimer's disease in the US population: Prevalence estimates using the 2000 Census. *Archives of Neurology* 60 (August 2003): 1119–1122.

Mathers, C., and M. Leonardi. Global burden of dementia in the year 2000: Summary of methods and data sources. Global Burden of Disease Project, World Health Organization, 2000.

Minino, A., M. Heron, S. Murphy, and K. Kochanek. Deaths Final Data for 2004. National Center for Health Statistics, Centers for Disease Control.

Skoog, I., and D. Gustafson. Update on hypertension and Alzheimer's disease. *Neurological Research* 28 (September 2006): 605–611.

Yaari, R., and J. Corey Bloom. Alzheimer's disease. *Seminars in Neurology* 27 (1): 32–41.

Chapter 3: Getting a Diagnosis

American Psychiatric Association. *DSM-IV-TR*. 2000.

Monien, B., L. Apostolova, and G. Bitan. Early diagnostics and therapeutics for Alzheimer's disease—how early can we get there? *Expert Reviews in Neurotherapeutics* 6 (9): 1293–1306.

Chapter 4: The Dementia Evaluation

Monnot, M., M. Brosey, and E. Ross. Screening for dementia: Family caregiver questionnaires reliably predict dementia. *Journal of the American Board of Family Practice* 18 (4): 240–256.

Chapter 5: Alzheimer's and Other Types of Dementia

Aggarwal, N., and C. DeCarli. Vascular dementia: Emerging trends. *Seminars in Neurology* 27 (1): 66–77.

Boeve, B. A review of the non-Alzheimer dementias. *Journal of Clinical Psychiatry* 67 (12): 1985–2001.

Clarfield, M. The decreasing prevalence of reversible dementias: an updated meta-analysis. *Archives of Internal Medicine* 163:2219–2229.

Graff-Radford, N., and B. Woodruff. Frontotemporal dementia. *Seminars in Neurology* 27 (1): 48–57.

Nitrini, R. The cure of one of the most frequent types of dementia: a historical parallel. *Alzheimer's Disease and Associated Disorder* 19 (3): 156–158.

Thompson, A., A. Peiper, and G. Treisman. Dementia and delirium in HIV-infected patients. Official reprint from UpToDate.

Weisman, D., and I. McKeith. Dementia with Lewy bodies. *Seminars in Neurology* 27 (1): 42–47.

Chapters 6 and 7: Treatments and Taking Care of the Whole Person

Aldridge, D., ed. *Music Therapy in Dementia Care*. London: Jessica Kingsley Publishers, 2000.

Birks, J., and J. Grimley Evans. Ginkgo biloba for cognitive impairment and dementia. Cochrane Database of Systematic Reviews 2007, Issue 2, Art. No. CD003120. DoI: 10.1002/14651858. CD003120.pub2

Diamond, B., S. Johnson, K. Torsney, J. Morodan, B. Prokop, D. Davidek, and P. Kramer. Complementary and alternative medicines in the treatment of dementia. *Drugs & Aging* 20 (13): 981–998.

Epperson, M., and W. Bonnel. Pain assessment in dementia: tools and strategies. *Clinical Excellence for Nurse Practitioners* 8 (4): 166–171.

Sierpina, V., B. Wollschlaeger, and M. Blumenthal. Ginkgo biloba. *American Family Physician* 68 (5).

Chapter 8: Medications

Beier, M. Treatment strategies for the behavioral symptoms of Alzheimer's disease: focus on early pharmacologic intervention. *Pharmacotherapy* 27 (3): 399–411.

Cummings, J. Alzheimer's disease. *New England Journal of Medicine* 351 (1): 56–67.

Chapter 9: Emotional and Behavioral Changes

Barak, Y., and D. Aizenber. Suicide amongst Alzheimer's disease patients: a 10-year study. *Dementia and Geriatric Cognitive Disorder* 14 (2002): 101–103.

Black, B., S. Muralee, and R. Tampi. Inappropriate sexual behaviors in dementia. *Journal of Geriatric Psychiatry and Neurology* 18 (3): 155–162.

Centers for Disease Control.. Nonfatal self-inflicted injuries among adults aged >65 years—United States 2005. *Morbidity and Mortality Weekly* 56 (38): 989–993.

Draper, B. Suicidal behavior in the elderly. *International Journal of Geriatric Psychiatry* 9 (January 1994): 655–661.

Draper, B., C. MacCuspie-Moore, and H. Brodaty. Suicidal ideation and the 'wish to die' in dementia patients: The role of depression. *Age and Ageing* 27 (4): 503–507.

McGonical-Kenney, M., and D. Schutte. Evidence-based guideline: Nonpharmacologic management of agitated behaviors in persons with Alzheimer's disease and other chronic dementing conditions. *Journal of Gerontological Nursing*, February 2006: 9–14.

Potter, G., and D. Steffens. Contribution of depression to cognitive impairment and dementia in older adults. *The Neurologist* 13 (3): 105–117.

Chapter 10: Keeping Your Loved One Safe

Carr, D., J. Duchek, T. Meuser, and J. Morris. Older adult drivers with cognitive impairment. *American Family Physician* 73 (6): 1029–1034.

Grabowski, D., C. Campbell, and M. Morrisey. Elderly licensure laws and motor vehicle fatalities. *JAMA* 291 (23): 2840–2846.

Odenheimer, G. Driver safety in older adults: The physician's role in assessing driving skill of older patients. *Geriatrics* 61 (10): 14–21.

Sherman, F. Driving: The ultimate IADL. *Geriatrics* 61 (10): 9–10.

Chapter 13: Advance Directives

American Health Insurance Plans. A Guide to Long-Term Care Insurance. 2003, 2004. Available through America's Health Insurance Plans (AHIP). 601 Pennsylvania Ave. NW, South Building, Suite 500, Washington, DC 20004. Tel: 202–778–3200, www.ahip.org.

Resnick, P. Competency and the law. *Audio-Digest Psychiatry* 36 (9).

Chapter 15: Nursing Homes and Extended-Care Facilities

Burger, S., V. Fraser, S. Hunt, and B. Frank. *Nursing Homes: Getting Good Care There.* 2nd ed. A consumer action manual prepared by The National Citizen's Coalition for Nursing Home Reform. Atascadero, CA: Impact Publishers, Inc., 2001.

Chapter 16: Caring for the Caregiver

Cannuscio, C., C. Jones, I. Kawachi, G. Colditz, L. Berkman, and E. Rimm. Reverberations of family illness: a longitudinal assessment of informal caregiving and mental health status in the Nurses' Health Study. *American Journal of Public Health* 92 (8): 1305–1311.

Gray, L. Caregiver depression: a growing mental health concern. Policy Brief, September 2003. Family Caregiver Alliance (National Center on Caregiving). www.caregiver.org

Loboprabhu, S., V. Molinari, and Lomax. *Supporting the Caregiver in Dementia: a Guide for Health Care Professionals.* Baltimore: The Johns Hopkins University Press, 2006.

U.S. Department of Health and Human Services/Administration on Aging. Caregiver Tip Sheet. Available at their web site: www.aoa.gov/prof/aoaprog/caregiver/overview/CaregiverTipSheet.pdf.

Chapter 19: Hope for the Future

Boche, D., J. Nicoll, and R. Weller. Immunotherapy for Alzheimer's disease and other dementias. *Current Opinion in Neurology* 18 (2005): 720–725.

Pollack, A. "Progress cited in Alzheimer's diagnosis. *The New York Times*, October 15, 2007.

RESOURCES

The Alzheimer's Association
National Office
225 N. Michigan Ave., Fl. 17
Chicago, IL 60601–7633
Tel: 312–335–8700
TTY: 312–335–5886
Fax: 866–699–1246
Website: www.alz.org

Administration on Aging (AOA)
Washington, DC 20201
Tel: 202–619–0724
Website: www.aoa.gov

The American Association of Retired Persons (AARP)
601 E Street NW
Washington, DC 20049
Tel: 888–687–2277
Website: www.aarp.org

American Health Care Association
1201 L Street NW
Washington, DC 20005
Tel: 202–842–4444
Website: www.ahcancal.org

The Hospice Foundation of America
Tel: 800–854–3402
Website: www.hospicefoundation.org

The Lewy Body Dementia Association, Inc.
P.O. Box 451429
Atlanta, GA 31145–9429
Helpline: 800–539–9767
Tel: 404–935–6444
Fax: 480–422–5434
Website: www.lewybodydementia.org

National Association of Estate Planners and Councils
1120 Chester Ave., Suite 470
Cleveland, OH 44114
Tel: 216–696–3225
Website: www.naepc.org

The National Citizen's Coalition for Nursing Home Reform
1828 L Street NW
Washington, DC 20036
Tel: 202–332–2275
Fax: 202–332–2949
Website: www.nccnhr.org

National Council on Aging
300 D Street, Suite 801
Washington, DC 20024
Tel: 202–479–1200
Website: www.ncoa.org

The National Family Caregiver Association (NFCA)
10400 Connecticut Avenue, Suite 500
Kensington, MD 20895–3944
Toll-Free: 800–896–3650
Tel: 301–942–6430
Fax: 301–942–2302
Website: www.nfcacares.org

The National Hospice and Palliative Care Association
Tel: 800–658–8898
Spanish help line: 877–658–8896
Website: www.caringinfo.org

Appendix C GERIATRIC QUESTIONNAIRE

(From the Personal History Questionnaire of the Dorothy Adler Geriatric Assessment Center at Yale-New Haven Hospital, New Haven, CT)

This questionnaire asks you for information that will help your treatment team answer your questions. This is a lengthy questionnaire, and the information you provide will allow for a more efficient visit. It's best to fill this out completely before going for your evaluation.

Today's date_____

Section 1

1. Patient's name:_____
2. Who filled out this form?_____
   a. Relationship if other than patient_____
   b. How often do you see the patient?_____
   c. Are you the caregiver most-involved with the patient?
      i.   _____YES
      ii.   _____NO → if NO, who is?_____
3. What are the most important questions or issues that you would like addressed at this evaluation?
   a.   _____

   _____

   _____

   b.   _____

   _____

   _____

   c.   _____

   _____

   _____

Section 2
General background questions

1. Is the patient currently (check one)
   a.   _____ Married?
   b.   _____ Divorced/Separated? When? _____
   c.   _____ Widowed? When? _____
   d.   _____ Single/Never married

e. _____ In a committed relationship/has a significant other?

f. _____ I'm not sure.

2. Please indicate the number of living close adult relatives the patient has:

   a. _____ Parents

   b. _____ Siblings (brothers and sisters)

   c. _____ Children

3. Please tell us about the patient's spouse and children from the current marriage, if any.

	Name	Age	Sex	City/State of residence	Telephone numbers
Spouse					
Children					

4. Please tell us about any children from prior marriages, if any.

	Name	Age	Sex	City/State of residence	Telephone numbers
Children					

5. Please tell us which close adult relatives live close to the patient (i.e., in the same state or in close driving or walking distance).

	Name	Relationship to patient	How often do they see the patient?
1.			
2.			
3.			
4.			
5.			
6.			
7.			

6. With whom does the patient live? (check all that apply)
    a. _____ Alone
    b. _____ With spouse or partner
    c. _____ With child/children or other family
    d. _____ Other, specify _____
    e. _____ I'm not sure

7. Which of the following best describes the patient's residence? (check one)
    a. _____ Own house or condo
    b. _____ Rental house, condo, or apartment
    c. _____ Lives with someone in their own home, condo, or apartment
    d. _____ Retirement community
    e. _____ Board and care/residential care facility/rest home/assisted-living
    f. _____ Nursing home/Skilled nursing facility/extended-care facility
    g. _____ Other, specify _____
    h. _____ I'm not sure

8. Where was the patient born?
    a. _____ State
    b. _____ Country

9. What is the patient's primary language?
    a. _____ English
    b. _____ Other language, specify _____

10. What is the patient's predominant ethnic origin?
    a. _____ Native American/American Indian

b. _____ Asian or Pacific Islander
c. _____ Black/African American
d. _____ Hispanic/Latino
e. _____ White/Caucasian
f. _____ Other, specify
g. _____ Not sure

11. What is the patient's religious preference or affiliation?

   _____

12. About how often does the patient go to religious meetings or services?
    a. _____ Never/almost never
    b. _____ Once or twice a year
    c. _____ Every few months
    d. _____ Once or twice a month
    e. _____ Weekly
    f. _____ More than once a week
    g. _____ I'm not sure

13. How much is religion a source of strength and comfort to the patient?
    a. _____ Not at all
    b. _____ A little
    c. _____ A great deal
    d. _____ I'm not sure

14. Education: What is the highest grade or year of regular school completed by the patient? (Please circle)

   Elementary School   0 1 2 3 4 5 6 7 8

High School   9 10 11 12
College   13 14 15 16 17 18 +

15. Work status. Is the patient currently: (check one)
    a.   _____Retired? If YES, how long? _____
    b.   _____ Working full-time
    c.   _____Working at least part-time
    d.   _____ Looking for work
    e.   _____ I'm not sure

16. What is, or was, the patient's principal occupation?
    _____

17. Is the patient a veteran of the armed forces?
    a.   _____ Yes
    b.   _____ No
    c.   _____ I'm not sure

18. How adequate do you think the patient's income is for his/her needs?
    a.   _____ Can't make ends meet.
    b.   _____ Has just enough money to make ends meet.
    c.   _____ Can comfortably meet financial needs.
    d.   _____ I'm not sure

19. Is there one person (family member or friend) who would make medical decisions for the patient if the patient couldn't make them for him/herself?
    a.   _____Yes → if YES, who? _____
    b.   _____ No
    c.   _____ I'm not sure

20. Has the patient designated a Durable Power of Attorney for finances and health care decisions?
    a. _____ Yes → if YES, who? _____
    b. _____ No
    c. _____ I'm not sure

21. Does the patient have a living will?
    a. _____ Yes → if YES, please bring a copy to the evaluation
    b. _____ No
    c. _____ I'm not sure

Section 3

This section asks about the patient's current abilities and needs, as well as the amount of support or help available to them.

	Without difficulty or help	With difficulty or needs some help	Completely unable to do on their own	I'm not sure
1. Can the patient feed him/ herself?				
2. Can the patient dress and undress?				
3. Can the patient take care of his/her own appearance (comb hair, brush teeth, etc.)?				
4. Can the patient walk?				
5. Can the patient get in and out of bed?				
6. Can the patient take a bath or shower?				

	Without difficulty or help	With difficulty or needs some help	Completely unable to do on their own	I'm not sure
7. Can the patient use the toilet?				
8. Can the patient use the telephone?				
9. Can the patient get to places out of walking distance by him/herself?				
10. Can the patient go shopping for groceries or clothes?				
11. Can the patient prepare his/her own meals?				
12. Can the patient do his/her own housework?				
13. Can the patient take his/her own medicines?				
14. Can the patient handle his/her own money?				

15. Can the patient walk half a mile (about eight blocks) without help?
    a. _____Yes
    b. _____ No
    c. _____ I'm not sure

16. Can the patient walk up and down stairs to the second floor without help?
   a. _____ Yes
   b. _____ No
   c. _____ I'm not sure

17. Does the patient currently participate in any regular activity or program designed to improve or maintain physical fitness?
   a. _____Yes → If yes, check what he/she does currently
      i.   ____Walking
      ii.   ____ Swimming
      iii. ____ Aerobics or exercise classes
      iv.   ____ Dancing
      v.   ____ Jogging
      vi.   ____ Bicycling or stationary bike
      vii. ____ Tennis
      viii. ____ Golf
      ix.   ____ Other specify: _____
   b. _____ No
   c. _____ I'm not sure

18. Does the patient drive a car?
   a. _____ Yes → If YES, is this a concern to you?
   i. _____ No
   ii. _____ Yes
   b. _____ No
   c. _____ I'm not sure

19. Do you have any safety concerns about the patient, other than driving (such as burning pots, tripping or falling, wandering, falling prey to criminals, or others)?
    a. _____Yes → If YES, please describe:

    _____

    _____
    b. _____ No
    c. _____ I'm not sure

20. Are there any guns in the patient's home?
    a. _____ Yes → If YES, please describe:

    _____

    _____
    b. _____ No
    c. _____ I'm not sure

21. Does the patient employ someone to provide care or help in the home?
    a. _____ Yes → If YES, how many hours a day and how many days a week is the paid helper available?
        i. _____ hours a day and _____ days a week
    b. _____ No
    c. _____ I'm not sure

22. Is this sufficient to meet the patient's needs?
    a. _____ Yes
    b. _____ No
    c. _____ I'm not sure

23. When the patient needs extra help with daily tasks, does he/she have anyone he/she can count on?
   a. _____Yes → If YES, who? _____
   b. _____ No
   c. _____ I'm not sure

24. Could the patient use more support with daily tasks than he/she has?
   a. _____ Yes
   b. _____ No
   c. _____ I'm not sure

25. Does the patient have anyone he/she can count on to provide emotional support, talking over problems, or helping make hard decisions?
   a. _____ Yes → If YES, who? _____
   b. _____ No
   c. _____ I'm not sure

26. Could the patient use more emotional support than he/she has?
   a. _____ Yes
   b. _____ No
   c. _____ I'm not sure

27. Does the patient provide care for a family member or significant other?
   a. _____Yes → If YES, who? _____
   b. _____ No
   c. _____ I'm not sure

28. How stressful do you, or others in the family, find it caring for the patient?
    a. _____ Not at all
    b. _____ Just a little bit
    c. _____ Quite a lot
    d. _____ Very much
    e. _____ I'm not sure

Section 4

This next section asks about common problems faced by older persons.

1. Do you have concerns about the patient's memory or ability to think clearly?
    a. _____ Yes
    b. _____ No
    c. _____ I'm not sure

2. Have you noticed any recent decline in the patient's ability to take care of household tasks or of him/herself?
    a. _____ Yes
    b. _____ No
    c. _____ I'm not sure

3. In the past month, has the patient been sad, blue, down in the dumps, or depressed?
    a. _____ Yes → if YES, has this been most of the day, nearly every day?
       i. _____ Yes
       ii. _____ No

b. _____ No

c. _____ I'm not sure

4. In the past month, has the patient been a lot less interested in most things, or unable to enjoy the things he/she used to enjoy?

a. _____ Yes → If YES, has this been most of the day, nearly every day?

    i. _____ Yes

    ii. _____ No

b. _____ No

c. _____ I'm not sure

5. Are you at all concerned about any of the patient's behavior, such as wandering, yelling, being aggressive, hostile, or suspicious, or seeing/hearing things that are not there?

a. _____ Yes → If YES, please describe

_____

_____

b. _____ No

c. _____ I'm not sure

6. Are you at all concerned about the patient's ability to get up and around on their own?

a. _____ Yes

b. _____ No

c. _____ I'm not sure

7. Has the patient had any falls in the past year?

a. _____ Yes → If YES, was he/she injured falling?

    i. _____ Yes

    ii. _____ No

b. _____ No

c. _____ I'm not sure

8. During the past 12 months has the patient ever lost his/her urine or gotten wet?
    a. _____ Yes → if YES, has this happened on at least six separate days?
        i. _____ Yes
        ii. _____ No
    b. _____ No
    c. _____ I'm not sure

9. Does the patient have a good appetite?
    a. _____ Yes
    b. _____ No
    c. _____ I'm not sure

10. Has the patient lost more than 10 pounds in the last 6 months?
    a. _____ Yes
    b. _____ No
    c. _____ I'm not sure

11. Does the patient wear glasses?
    a. _____ Yes
    b. _____ No
    c. _____ I'm not sure

12. Has the patient seen an eye specialist (Optometrist, Ophthalmologist) in the past year?
    a. _____ Yes
    b. _____ No

c. _____ I'm not sure

13. Do you think the patient has problems hearing?
    a. _____ Yes → If YES, does he/she wear a hearing aid(s)?
        i. _____ Yes
        ii. _____ No
    b. _____ No
    c. _____ I'm not sure

14. As far as you know, is difficulty sleeping interfering with the patient's quality of life?
    a. _____ Yes → If YES, which of the following problems does the patient have? (check all that apply)
        i. _____ Trouble falling asleep
        ii. _____ Trouble falling back asleep after waking at night
        iii. _____ Waking up too early in the morning
        iv. _____ Sleepiness during the daytime
        v. _____ A lot of snoring
        vi. _____ Something else, describe:

_____

_____

    b. _____ No
    c. _____ I'm not sure

15. Does the patient drink alcohol, including beer and wine?
    a. _____ Yes → If YES, how often
        i. _____ daily
        ii. _____ Greater than 3 times per week
        iii. _____ 1 to 3 times per week
        iv. _____ Less than 1 time a week
    b. _____ No

c. _____ I'm not sure

16. Does the patient drink to the point of becoming drunk, passing out, or blacking out?
    a. _____ Yes → If YES, How often does this happen?

    _____

    _____

    b. _____ No
    c. _____ I'm not sure

17. Do you think the patient has a problem with drugs or alcohol?
    a. _____ Yes → If yes, Please describe:

    _____

    _____

    b. _____ No
    c. _____ I'm not sure

18. Does the patient currently smoke?
    a. _____ Yes
    b. _____ No → If NO, is the patient a former smoker?
       i. _____ Yes
       ii. _____ No
    c. _____ I'm not sure

Section 5

This final section asks about the patient's health and medical history. Please answer the questions to the best of your knowledge.

1. Which medical conditions does the patient have now or has the patient had in the past? (check all that apply)

Eye & Ear Problems	Check if Yes	Kidney and Urinary Tract Problems	Check if Yes
Cataracts		Kidney disease	
Glaucoma		Prostate disease	
Macular degeneration of the eye		Frequent bladder or kidney infections	
Hearing Loss/Hearing aid		Other (Specify)	
Other (specify)		Gastrointestinal Problems	
Heart Problems		Ulcers	
Angina		Heartburn	
Heart attack		Hiatal hernia	
Heart Failure (CHF)		Diverticulosis	
High Blood Pressure/ Hypertension		Liver Disease/Cirrhosis	
Irregular Heart beats		Hepatitis	
Other (specify)		Polyps	
Lung Problems		Gallbladder Disease	
Asthma		Other (specify)	
Bronchitis		Nervous System Problems	
Emphysema		Stroke	
Other (Specify)		Dementia/Alzheimer's disease	
Bone and Joint Problems		Parkinson's disease	
Arthritis		Epilepsy/Seizures	
Osteoporosis (fragile bones)		Other (Specify)	
Fractured hip, wrist or spine (circle which one)		Other Health Problems	
Gout		Anemia	

...Continued

Eye & Ear Problems	Check if Yes	Kidney and Urinary Tract Problems	Check if Yes
Other (Specify)		Blood clots	
		Cancer (specify type)	
		Depression	
		Other psychiatric problems	
		Sexual function problems	
		Other (Specify)	

2. List any surgeries (operations) the patient has had. Attach another page if needed.

Date	Surgery (Operation)

3. List any other hospitalization the patient has had. Start with the most recent. Attach another page if needed.

Date	Reason

4. To be certain everything is covered, please indicate whether, to the best of your knowledge, the patient has had any of the following symptoms or problems during the last three months (check all that apply).

Eye & Ear Problems	Check if Yes	Kidney and Urinary Tract Problems	Check if Yes
Visual or eye problems		Urination at night	
Hearing difficulty or ear trouble		Frequent urination	
Heart Problems		Painful urination	
Chest pain or tightness		Difficulty starting or stopping urination	
Rapid or irregular heart beat		Frequent accidents	

...Continued

Eye & Ear Problems	Check if Yes	Kidney and Urinary Tract Problems	Check if Yes
Lung Problems		Brain and Nervous System Problems	
Persistent cough		Frequent headaches	
Difficulty breathing or shortness of breath		Frequent dizzy spells	
Digestion Problems		Passing out or fainting	
Dental/Teeth problems		Paralysis, leg or arm weakness	
Difficulty swallowing		Numbness or loss of feeling	
Frequent indigestion/stomach ache		Serious problems with memory, or difficulty thinking	
Nausea and vomiting		Tremor or shaking	
Change in bowel habits		Gynecology Problems	
Weight loss (how much?)		Vaginal bleeding after menopause	
Black bowel movements or blood from the rectum		Breast lumps or discomfort	
Frequent diarrhea		Vaginal discharge	
Persistent constipation		Other Health Problems	
Bone and Joint Problems		Difficulty with sleeping	
Leg pain on walking		Swelling of feet or ankles	
Back or neck pain		Fever	
Joint paint or stiffness		Excessive sweating	
Foot problems		Other:	

_____ Check here if he/she has not had any of these problems in the last 3 months.

5. Please list the patient's current medications, both prescription and over-the-counter, and include the dosage and frequency of their use. Note: It's also a very good idea to bring all medications in their original bottles to your evaluation.

	Medication	Dosage (How many milligrams)	Frequency (How many times a day)	Prescribed by
1				
2				
3				
4				
5				
6				
7				
8				
9				
10				
11				
12				
13				
14				
15				
16				
17				
18				
19				

6. Patient's Pharmacy (please include phone number):

   _____

   _____

   _____

7. Patient's Physician(s)
   a. Internist or primary care physician (please include phone number):

      _____

      _____

      _____

   b. Specialists (please include type of specialty and phone number)
      i.   _____

           _____

           _____

      ii. _____

           _____

           _____

      iii. _____

           _____

           _____

Is there anything else you think it's important that the evaluation professional or team knows? Please describe it below, or make a note to discuss it at the evaluation. Thank you.

Appendix D

STATE	State Commission and/or Agency on Aging	State Long-Term Care Ombudsman
Alabama	Alabama Department of Senior Services 770 Washington Avenue RSA Plaza Suite 470 Montgomery, AL 36130 Tel: 334–242–5743 Toll-free: 877–425–2243 Website: http://www.adss.state.al.us To find your local Agency on Aging: Tel: 800-AGELINE (800–243–5463) Fax: 334–242–5594 Email: ageline@adss.alabama.gov Website: http://www.adss.state.al.us/aaa.cfm	Alabama Long Term Care Ombudsman Department of Senior Services 770 Washington Avenue RSA Plaza Building, Suite 470 Montgomery, AL 36130 Tel: 334–242–5770 Fax: 334–353–8467 Website: www.ageline.gov

Alaska	State of Alaska Department of Health and Human Services Senior and Disabilities Services 240 Main Street, Suite 601 Juneau, AK 99811–0680 Tel: 907–465–3372 Toll-free: 866–465–3165 TTY: 907–465–5430 Fax: 907- 465–1170 Website: www.hss.state.ak.us/dsds **Alaska Commission on Aging** Alaska Department of Health & Social Services P. O. Box 110693 Juneau, AK 99811–0693 Tel: 907–465–3250 Fax: 907–465–1398 Website: www.hss.state.ak.us/acoa	**Alaska Mental Health Trust Authority** Office of the State Long Term Care Ombudsman 3745 Community Park Loop, Suite 200 Anchorage, AK 99508 Tel: 907–334–4480 Fax: 907–334–4486 Website: www.akoltco.org
Arizona	**Aging and Adult Administration** Department of Economic Security 1789 W Jefferson St., #950A Phoenix, AZ 85007 Tel: 602–542–4446 Fax: 602–542–6575 Website with locator for regional offices: www.azdes.gov/aaa/regions/default.asp	**State Long-Term Care Ombudsman** Arizona Department of Economic Security Div. of Aging and Adult Services 1789 W Jefferson St., #950A Phoenix, AZ 85007 Tel: 602–542–6440

Arkansas	**Division of Aging & Adult Services** Arizona Department of Human Services P. O. Box 1437, Slot 1412 Little Rock, AR 72203–1437 Tel: 501–682–2441 Fax: 501–682–8155 Website with directory of services: www.arkansas.gov/dhs/aging/ agedrcty.html	**State Long-Term Care Ombudsman** Arizona Division of Aging & Adult Services P. O. Box 1437, Slot S-540 Little Rock, AR 72203 Tel: 501–682–8952 Fax: 501–682–6393
California	**Department of Aging** California Department of Aging 1300 National Drive, Suite 200 Sacramento, CA 95834 Tel: 916–419–7500 Fax: 916–928–2267 Website: www.aging.ca.gov This includes links to area resources and agencies on aging.	**State Long-Term Care Ombudsman** California Department of Aging 1300 National Drive, Suite 200 Sacramento, CA 95834 Tel: 916–419–7510 Fax: 916–928–2503 Website: www.aging.ca.gov/html/ programs/ombudsman.html
Colorado	**Division of Aging and Adult Services** Department of Human Services 1575 Sherman Street, 10th Floor Denver, CO 80203–1714 Tel: 303–866–2800 Fax: 303–866–4214 Web site: www.cdhs.state.co.us/ aas/index.htm	**State Long-Term Care Ombudsman** The Legal Center 455 Sherman Street, Suite 130 Denver, CO 80203 Tel: 800–288–1376 Fax: 303–722–0720 Website: www.thelegalcenter.org/ services_older.html

Connecticut	Department of Social Services Elderly Services Division 25 Sigourney St., 10th Floor Hartford, CT 06106–5033 Tel: 860–424–5277 Fax: 860–424–5301 Website: www.ct.gov/agingservices/site/default.asp	State Long-Term Care Ombudsman Connecticut Department of Social Services Office of the State Long Term Care Ombudsman 25 Sigourney Street, 12th Floor, Hartford, CT 06106–5033 Tel: 860–424–5238 Fax: 860–424–4808 Website: www.ltcop.state.ct.us
Delaware	Delaware Division of Services for Aging & Adults with Physical Disabilities Dept. of Health and Social Services 1901 North Dupont Highway New Castle, DE 19720 Tel: 302–255–9390 Fax: 302–255–4445 Website: www.dhss.delaware.gov/dsaapd	State Long-Term Care Ombudsman Division of Services for Aging & Adults 1901 North Dupont Highway Main Admin. Bldg. Annex New Castle, DE 19720 Tel: 302–255–9390 Fax: 302–255–4445 Website: www.dhss.delaware.gov/dsaapd Link for program specifics: www.dhss.delaware.gov/dhss/dsaapd/ltcop.html
District of Columbia	DC Office on Aging One Judiciary Square 441 4th Street NW, Suite 900 Washington, DC 20001 Tel: 202–724–5622 Fax: 202–724–4979 Website: www.dcoa.dc.gov/dcoa/site/default.asp	State Long-Term Care Ombudsman 601 E Street NW, A4–315 Washington, DC 20049 Tel: 202–434–2140 Fax: 202–434–6595 Website: www.aarp.org/states/dc/dc-lce/a2003-05-08-lce_longtermcare.html

Florida	**Florida Department of Elder Affairs** Building B, Suite 152 4040 Esplanade Way Tallahassee, FL 32399–7000 Tel: 850–414–2000 Fax: 850–414–2004 Website: www.elderaffairs.state.fl.us	**State Long-Term Care Ombudsman** Florida State Long Term Care Ombudsman Council Department of Elder Affairs 4040 Esplanade Way Tallahassee, FL 32399 Tel: 888–831–0404 Fax: 850–414–2377 Website: www.myflorida.com/ombudsman
Georgia	**Georgia Division of Aging Services** Department of Human Resources 2 Peachtree St. NW, 9th Floor Atlanta, GA 30303–3142 Tel: 404–657–5252 Fax: 404–657–5285 Website: www.aging.dhr.georgia.gov/portal/site	**State Long-Term Care Ombudsman** Office of the State Long Term Care Ombudsman 2 Peachtree St. NW, 9th Floor Atlanta, GA 30303–3142 Tel: 888–454–5826 Fax: 404–463–8384 Website: www.georgiaombudsman.org
Hawaii	**Hawaii Executive Office on Aging** Number 1 Capitol District 250 South Hotel St., Suite 109 Honolulu, HI 96813–2831 Tel: 808–586–0100 Fax: 808–586–0185 Website: www4.hawaii.gov/eoa/	**State Long-Term Care Ombudsman** Executive Office on Aging 250 South Hotel St., Suite 406 Honolulu, HI 96813–2831 Tel: 808–586–0100 Fax: 808–586–0185 Website: www2.state.hi.us/eoa/

Idaho	Idaho Commission on Aging P. O. Box 83720 3380 Americana Terrace, Suite 120 Boise, ID 83720–0007 Tel: 208–334–3833 Toll-free: 877–471–2777 Website: www.idahoaging.com/ abouticoa/index.htm	State Long-Term Care Ombudsman Idaho Commission on Aging P. O. Box 83720 3380 American Terrace, Suite 120 Boise, ID 83720–0007 Tel: 208–334–3833 Fax: 208–334–3033 Website: www.idahoaging.com/ programs/ps_ombuds.htm
Illinois	Illinois Department on Aging 421 East Capitol Ave., #100 Springfield, IL 62701–1789 Tel: 217–785–3356 Fax: 217–785–4477 Website: www.state.il.us/aging/	State Long-Term Care Ombudsman Illinois Department on Aging 421 East Capitol Avenue, Suite 100 Springfield, IL 62701–1789 Tel: 217–785–3143 Fax: 217–524–9644 Website: www.state.il.us/aging
Indiana	Bureau of Aging and In-Home Services 402 W Washington St., #W454 P. O. Box 7083 Indianapolis, IN 46207–7083 Tel: 317–232–7020 Fax: 317–232–7867 Website: www.in.gov/fssa/da/index.htm	State Long-Term Care Ombudsman Indiana Division of Disabilities and Rehabilitation Services 402 W. Washington St., #W 454 P. O. Box 7083, MS21 Indianapolis, IN 46207–7083 Tel: 800–622–4484 Fax: 317–232–7867

Iowa	**Iowa Department of Elder Affairs** Jessie M. Parker Building 510 E 12th Street, Suite 2 Des Moines, IA 50319 Tel: 515–725–3301 Fax: 515–725–3300 Website: www.iowa.gov/elderaffairs/	**State Long-Term Care Ombudsman** Iowa Department of Elder Affairs Jessie M. Parker Bldg 510 E 12th Street, Suite 2 Des Moines, IA 50319 Tel: 515–725–3327 Fax: 515–725–3300 Website: www.iowa.gov/elderaffairs/advocacy/ombudsman.html
Kansas	**Kansas Department on Aging** New England Building 503 South Kansas Avenue Topeka, KS 66603 Tel: 785–296–4986 Toll-free: 800–432–3535 TTY: 785–291–3167 Fax: 785–296–0256 Website: www.agingkansas.org/	**State Long-Term Care Ombudsman** Office of the State Long Term Care Ombudsman 900 SW Jackson Street, Suite 1041 Topeka, KS 66612 Tel: 877–662–8362 Toll-free (Kansas only): 877–662–8362 Fax: 785–296–3916 Website: http://da.ks.gov/care
Kentucky	**Cabinet for Health & Family Services** Division of Aging Services 275 East Main Street, 3W-F Frankfort, KY 40621 Tel: 502–564–6930 Fax: 502–564–4595 Website: http://chfs.ky.gov/ Link to area agencies on aging: www.kentucky.gov/Portal/Search.aspx	**State Long-Term Care Ombudsman** Cabinet for Health & Family Services Office of the Ombudsman 275 East Main Street, 1E-B Frankfort, KY 40621 Tel: 502–564–5497 Toll-free: 800–372–2973 TTY: 800–627–4702 Fax: 502–564–9523 Website: http://chfs.ky.gov/omb/

Louisiana	Governor's Office on Elderly Affairs 412 N 4th Street, 3rd Floor Baton Rouge, LA 70802 Tel: 225–342–7100 Fax: 225–342–7133 Website: http://goea.louisiana.gov/ index.html **Council on Aging** P. O. Box 1482 824 East 1st Street Crowley, LA 70527 Tel: 337–788–1400 Fax: 337–788–3198 Website: http://goea.louisiana.gov/ council_on_aging.html	State Long-Term Care Ombudsman Office of Elderly Affairs 412 N 4th Street, 3rd Floor P. O. Box 61 Baton Rouge, LA 70821 Tel: 866–632–0922 Fax: 225–342–7144 Website: http://goea.louisiana.gov/ LTC_ombudsman.html
Maine	**Department of Health and Human Services (Office of Elder Services)** Maine Health and Human Services 11 State House Station 442 Civic Center Drive Augusta, ME 04333 Tel: 207–287–9200 Toll-free: 800–262–2232 TTY: 800–606–0215 Fax: 207–287–9229 Website: www.maine.gov/dhhs/beas/	State Long-Term Care Ombudsman 1 Weston Court P. O. Box 128 Augusta, ME 04332 Tel: 207–621–1079 Fax: 207–621–0509 Website: www.maineombudsman.org

Maryland	**Maryland Department of Aging** State Office Bldg., Room 1007 301 W Preston Street Baltimore, MD 21201–2374 Tel: 410–767–1100 Fax: 410–333–7943 Website: www.mdoa.state.md.us/	**State Long-Term Care Ombudsman** Maryland Department of Aging State Office Bldg., Room 1007 301 W Preston Street Baltimore, MD 21201–2374 Tel: 410–767–1100 Fax: 410–333–7943 Website: www.mdoa.state. md.us/ombudsman.html
Massachusetts	**Massachusetts Executive Office of Elder Affairs** One Ashburton Place, 5th Floor Boston, MA 02108 Tel: 617–727–7750 Fax: 617–727–6944 Website: www.mass.gov/?pageID= eldershomepage&L=1&L0= Home&sid= Elders	**State Long-Term Care Ombudsman** Massachusetts Executive Office of Elder Affairs 1 Ashburton Place, 5th Floor Boston, MA 02108–1518 Tel: 617–727–7750 Fax: 617–727–9368 Website: www.mass.gov/?pageID= elderstopic&L=3&L0=Home&L1= Service+Organizations+and+ Advocates&L2=Long+Term+ Care+Ombudsman&sid=Elders

Michigan	**Michigan Office of Services to the Aging** 7109 West Sagninaw, 1st Floor P.O. Box 30676 Lansing, MI 48909–8176 Tel: 517–373–7876 Fax: 517–373–4092 Website: ww.michigan.gov/miseniors	**State Long-Term Care Ombudsman** Michigan Office of Services to the Aging 7109 West Saginaw P. O. Box 30676 Lansing, MI 48909–8176 Tel: 517–335–0148 Toll-free: 866–485–9393 Fax: 517–373–4092 Website: http://www.michigan.gov/miseniors/0,1607,7–234–43230_46224—,00.html
Minnesota	**Minnesota Board on Aging** P. O. Box 64976 St. Paul, MN 55164–0976 Tel: 651–431–2565 Fax: 651–431–7415 Website: www.mnaging.org./ Minnesota Association of Area Agencies on Aging Senior LinkAge Line: 800–333–2433 Website: www.minnesota-aaa.org/	**Office of Ombudsman for Older Minnesotans** P. O. Box 64971 St. Paul, MN 55164–0971 Tel: 651–431–2604 Fax: 651–431–7452 Website: www.mnaging.org./admin/ooom.htm
Mississippi	**Mississippi Department of Human Services/Division of Aging and Adult Services** Council on Aging 750 North State Street Jackson, MS 39202 Tel: 601–359–4925 Fax: 601–359–9664 Website: www.mdhs.state.ms.us/aas.html Website for Area Agencies on Aging: www.mdhs.state.ms.us/aas_agcy.html	**State Long-Term Care Ombudsman** Mississippi Department of Human Services, Division of Aging 750 North State Street Jackson, MS 39202 Tel: 601–359–4927 Fax: 601–359–9664

Missouri	**Department of Health and Senior Services** P. O. Box 570 Jefferson City, MO 65102 Tel: 573–751–6400 Fax: 573–751–6041 Website: www.dhss.mo.gov/index.html	**State Long-Term Care Ombudsman** Department of Health & Senior Services P. O. Box 570 Jefferson City, MO 65102 Tel: 800–309–3282 Fax: 573–751–6499 Website: www.dhss.mo.gov/ Ombudsman/
Montana	**Senior and Long Term Care Division/Department of Public Health and Human Services** P. O. Box 4210 111 N Sanders, Room 211 Helena, MT 59604 Tel: 406–444–7788 Fax: 406–444–7743 Website: www.dphhs.mt.gov/ index.shtml	**State Long-Term Care Ombudsman** Montana Department of Health & Human Services P. O. Box 4210 111 N Sanders Helena, MT 59604–4210 Tel: 406–444–7785 Toll-free: 800–332–2272 Fax: 406–444–7743 Website: www.dphhs.mt.gov/ sltc/services/aging/ ltcombudsman.shtml
Nebraska	**Nebraska Department of Health and Human** Services/State Unit on Aging P. O. Box 95026 Lincoln, NE 68509–5044 Tel: 402- 471–4623 Toll-free: 800–942–7830 (Nebraska only) Fax: 402–471–4619 Website: www.hhs.state.ne.us/ags/ agsindex.htm	**State Long-Term Care Ombudsman** Division of Aging Services State Unit on Aging P. O. Box 95026 Lincoln, NE 68509–5044 Tel: 402–471–2307 Fax: 402–471–4619 Website: http://www.hhs.state. ne.us/ags/ltcombud.htm

| Nevada | Division for Aging Services/State of Nevada Department of Health and Human Services Carson City 3416 Goni Rd., Bldg D, Suite 132 Carson City, NV 89706 Tel: 775–687–4210 Fax: 775–687–4264 Las Vegas 3100 W Sahara Ave, Suite 103 Las Vegas, NV 89102 Tel: 702–486–3545 Fax: 702–486–3572 Elko 850 Elm Street Elko, NV 89801 Tel: 775–738–1966 Fax: 775–753–8543 Reno 445 Apple Street, Suite 104 Reno, NV 89502 Tel: 775–688–2964 Fax: 775–688–2969 Website: www.nvaging.net/ | State Long-Term Care Ombudsman Nevada Division for Aging Services 3100 W Sahara Ave., Suite 115 Las Vegas, NV 89102 Tel: 702–486–3545 Fax: 702–486–3572 Website: www.nvaging.net/ltc.htm |
| New Hampshire | Department of Health and Human Services/Bureau of Elderly and Adult Services 129 Pleasant St. Concord, NH 03301–3852 Tel: 603–271–4680 Website: www.dhhs.state.nh.us/DHHS/BEAS/default.htm | New Hampshire Office of the Long-Term Care Ombudsman 129 Pleasant Street Concord, NH 03301–3857 Tel: 603–271–4704 Fax: 603–271–5574 Website: www.dhhs.state.nh.us/DHHS/OLTCO/default.htm |

New Jersey	**New Jersey Division of Aging & Community Services** Department of Health & Senior Services P. O. Box 807 Trenton, NJ 08625–0807 Tel: 609–943–3345 Fax: 609–943–3343 Website: www.state.nj.us/health/senior/	**Office of Ombudsman for the Institutionalized Elderly** P. O. Box 807 Trenton, NJ 08625–0852 Tel: 609–943–3451 Toll-free: 877–582–6995 Fax: 609–943–3479 Website: www.state.nj.us/ publicadvocate/seniors/elder/
New Mexico	**New Mexico Aging & Long Term Care Services Department** Toney Anaya Building 2550 Cerrillos Road Sante Fe, NM 87505 Tel: 505–476–4799 Toll-free: 866–451–2901 (New Mexico only) Fax: 505–827–7649 Website: www.nmaging.state.nm.us/	**State Long-Term Care Ombudsman** New Mexico Aging & Long Term Care Services Dept. 2550 Cerrillos Road Santa Fe, NM 87505 Tel: 505–476–4790 Fax: 505–476–4836 Website: www.nmaging.state.nm.us/ Ombudsman_bureau.html
New York	**New York State Office for the Aging** 2 Empire State Plaza Albany, NY 12223–1251 Tel: 518–474–7012 Toll-free: 800–342–9871 (New York only) Fax: 518–474–1398 Website: http://aging.state.ny.us/	**State Long-Term Care Ombudsman** New York State Office for the Aging 2 Empire State Plaza Agency Building #2 Albany, NY 12223 Tel: 518–474–7329 Toll-free: 1–800–342–9871 (New York only) Fax: 518–474–7761 Website: www.ombudsman.state.ny.us/

North Carolina	**North Carolina Division of Aging and Adult Services** 2101 Mail Service Center Raleigh, NC 27699–2101 Tel: 919 733–3983 Fax: 919–733–0443 Website: www.ncdhhs.gov/aging/index.htm	**State Long-Term Care Ombudsman** North Carolina Division of Aging & Adult Services Long-Term Care Ombudsman Program 2101 Mail Service Center Raleigh, NC 27699–2101 Tel: 919–733–8395 Fax: 919–715–0868 Website: www.dhhs.state.nc.us/aging/ombud.htm
North Dakota	**North Dakota Department of Human Services/Adults and Aging Services** 600 E Boulevard Ave., Dept 325 Bismarck, ND 58505–0250 Tel: 701–328–4601 TTY: 701–328–3480 Fax: 701- 328–4061 Senior Infoline: 800–451–8693 Website: www.nd.gov/dhs/services/adultsaging/index.html	**Long-Term Care Ombudsman Program** 1237 West Divide Avenue, Suite 6 Bismarck, ND 58501 Tel: 800–451–8693 Fax: 701–328–8744 Website: www.nd.gov/dhs/services/adultsaging/ombudsman.html
Ohio	**Ohio Department of Aging** 50 W Broad St., 9th Floor Columbus, OH 43215–3363 Tel: 800–266–4346 TTY: 614–466–6191 Website: www.goldenbuckeye.com/	**State Long-Term Care Ombudsman** Ohio Department of Aging 50 W Broad Street, 9th Floor Columbus, OH 43215–3363 Tel: 614–644–7922 Fax: 614–644–5201 Website: http://goldenbuckeye.com/families/ombudsman.html

Oklahoma	**Aging Services Division** Department of Human Services 2401 NW 23rd Street, Suite 40 Oklahoma City, OK 73107 Tel: 405–521–2327 Senior Infoline: 800–211–2116 Fax: 405–521–2086 Website: www.okdhs.org/ programsandservices/docs/ olderoklahomans.htm	**State Long-Term Care Ombudsman** Department of Human Services/Aging Services Division 2401 NW 23rd Street, Suite 40 Oklahoma City, OK 73107 Tel: 405–521–6734 Fax: 405–522–6739 Website: www.okdhs.org/ programsandservices/aging/ltc/
Oregon	**Seniors and People with Physical Disabilities Division** Oregon Department of Human Services 500 Summer St. NE, E 02 Salem, OR 97301–1002 Tel: 503–945–5858 Fax: 503–373–7823 Website: www.oregon.gov/DHS/ spwpd/index.shtml	**State Long-Term Care Ombudsman** 3855 Wolverine NE, Suite 6 Salem, OR 97305–1251 Tel: 503–378–6533 Fax: 503–373–0852 Website: www.oregon.gov/ltco
Pennsylvania	**Pennsylvania Department of Aging** 555 Walnut Street, 5th Floor Harrisburg, PA 17101–1919 Tel: 717–783–7096 Fax: 717–783–6842 Email: aging@state.pa.us Website: www.aging.state.pa.us/aging/ site/default.asp Pennsylvania Council on Aging Tel: 717–783–1924	**State Long-Term Care Ombudsman** Pennsylvania Department of Aging 555 Walnut Street, 5th Floor P. O. Box 1089 Harrisburg, PA 17101 Tel: 717–783–7096 Toll-free: 877–724–3258 (Pennsylvania only) Fax: 717–772–3382 Website: www.dsf.health.state.pa. us/health/cwp/view.asp?A=188& Q=200735

Puerto Rico	**Puerto Rico Governor's Office of Elder Affair** P. O. Box 191179 San Juan, PR 00919–1179 Tel: 787–725–1515 Toll-free: 877–725–4300 Fax: 787–721–6510	State Long-Term Care Ombudsman Puerto Rico Governor's Office of Elder Affair P. O. Box 191179 San Juan, PR 00919–1179 Tel: 787–725–1515 Fax: 787–721–6510
Rhode Island	**Rhode Island Department of Elderly Affairs** John O. Pastore Center 35 Howard Ave., 2nd Floor Benjamin Rush Bldg., #55 Cranston, RI 02920 Tel: 401–462–0501 Fax: 401–462–0503 Website: www.dea.state.ri.us/	State Long-Term Care Ombudsman Alliance for Better Long Term Care 422 Post Road, Suite 204 Warwick, RI 02888 Tel 401–785–3340 Fax: 401–785–3391
South Carolina	**Governor's Office on Aging** 1301 Gervais Street, Suite 200 Columbia, SC 29201 Tel: 803–734–9898 Fax: 803–734–9986 Website: www.aging.sc.gov	State Long-Term Care Ombudsman Governor's Office on Aging 1301 Gervais Street, Suite 200 Columbia, SC 29201 Tel: 803–734–9898 Fax: 803–734–9986 Website: www.aging.sc.gov/ Seniors/Ombudsman.htm
South Dakota	**Office of Adult Services & Aging/Department of Social Services** 700 Governor's Drive Pierre, SD 57501–2291 Tel: 605–773–3656 Fax: 605–773–6834 Website: http://dss.sd.gov/elderlyservices /index.asp	State Long-Term Care Ombudsman South Dakota Office of Adult Services & Aging Department of Social Services 700 Governors Drive Pierre, SD 57501–2291 Tel: 605–773–3656 Toll-free: 866–854–5465 Fax: 605–773–6834 Website: http://dss.sd.gov/elderlyservices/ services/ombudsman.asp

Tennessee	Tennessee Commission on Aging and Disability Andrew Jackson Bldg. 500 Deaderick Street, Ste. 825 Nashville, TN 37243 Tel: 615–741–2056 Fax: 615–741–3309 Website: www.state.tn.us/comaging/	State Long-Term Care Ombudsman Tennessee Commission on Aging and Disability Andrew Jackson Bldg. 500 Deaderick Street, Ste. 825 Nashville, TN 37243 Tel: 615–741–2056 ext. 122 Toll-free: 877–236–0013 TTY: 615–532–3893 Fax: 615–741–3309 Website: www.state.tn.us/comaging/ombudsman.html
Texas	Texas Department of Aging and Disability Services John H. Winters Human Services Complex 701 W 51st St. P.O. Box 149030 Austin, TX 78714–9030 Tel: 512–438–3011 Fax: 512–438–4747 Website: www.dads.state.tx.us/	State Long-Term Care Ombudsman Center for Consumer and External Affairs P. O. Box 149030 Mail Code 250 Austin, TX 78714 Tel: 512–438–4356 Fax: 512–438–3223 Website: www.dads.state.tx.us/news_info/ombudsman/index.html
Utah	Utah Division of Aging & Adult Services Department of Human Services 120 North 200 West, Room 325 Salt Lake City, UT 84103 Tel: 801–538–3924 Fax: 801–538–4395 Website: www.hsdaas.utah.gov/	State Long-Term Care Ombudsman Utah Division of Aging & Adult Services Department of Human Services 120 North 200 West, Room 325 Salt Lake City, UT 84103 Tel: 801–538–3924 Toll-free: 800–662–4157 Fax: 801–538–4395 Website: www.hsdaas.utah.gov/ltco_about.htm

Vermont	Vermont Department of Disabilities, Aging and Independent Living/Division of Disability and Aging Services Waterbury Complex 103 South Main Street Waterbury, VT 05671–2301 Tel: 802–241–2400 Fax: 802–241–2325 Website: http://dail.vermont.gov/ To find your local Area Agency on Aging: www.dad.state.vt.us/dail/Guidetoservices/government/major.htm	State Long-Term Care Ombudsman Vermont Legal Aid, Inc. 264 N. Winooski Avenue P. O. Box 1367 Burlington, VT 05402 Tel: 802–863–5620 Fax: 802–863–7152 Website: www.dad.state.vt.us/ltcinfo/ombudsman.html
Virginia	Virginia Department for the Aging 1610 Forest Avenue, Suite 100 Richmond, VA 23229 Tel: 804–662–9333 Toll-free: 800–552–3402 Fax: 804–662–9354 Website: www.vda.virginia.gov/	State Long-Term Care Ombudsman Virginia Association of Area Agencies on Aging 24 E. Cary Street, Suite 100 Richmond, VA 23219 Tel: 804–565–1600 Fax: 804–644–5640 Website: www.vaaaa.org
Washington	Department of Social and Health Services/Aging and Disability Services Administration 640 Woodland Square Loop Lacey, WA 98503 Tel: 360–902–7797 Fax: 360–902–7848 Website: www.aasa.dshs.wa.gov/	State Long-Term Care Ombudsman Multi-Service Center 1200 S 336th Street P. O. Box 23699 Federal Way, WA 98093 Tel: 800–422–1384 Fax: 253–815–8173 Website: www.ltcsop.org

West Virginia	West Virginia Bureau of Senior Services 1900 Kanawha Boulevard East Bldg #10 Charleston, WV 25305–0160 Tel: 304–558–3317 Fax: 304–558–0004 Website: www.state. wv.us/ seniorservices/	State Long-Term Care Ombudsman West Virginia Bureau of Senior Services 1900 Kanawha Boulevard East Bldg #10 Charleston, WV 25305–0160 Tel: 304–558–3317 Toll-free: 800–834–0598 Fax: 304–558–0004 Website: www.wvseniorservices.gov/ wvboss_article2.cfm?atl=ACE1FD0C-D1FE-11D5–8DA00002A52CB920& fs=1 (or just enter the word "ombudsman" into the search box of the bureau's website)
Wisconsin	Wisconsin Board on Aging & Long Term Care 1402 Pankratz St., Suite 111 Madison, WI 53704–4001 Tel: 715–582–0124 Fax: 920–492–5951 Website: http://longtermcare. state.wi.us	State Long-Term Care Ombudsman Wisconsin Board on Aging & Long Term Care 1402 Pankratz Street, Suite 111 Madison, WI 53704–4001 Tel: 715–582–0124 Toll-free: 1–800–815–0015 Fax: 920–492–5951 Website: http://longtermcare.state.wi.us/ home/Ombudsman.htm
Wyoming	Wyoming Department of Health/Division on Aging 6101 Yellow Stone Rd., #259B Cheyenne, WY 82002–0710 Tel: 307–777–7986 Fax: 307–777–5340 Website: http://wdhfs.state. wy.us/aging/index.html	State Long-Term Care Ombudsman Wyoming Senior Citizens, Inc 865 Gilchrist, P. O. Box 94 Wheatland, WY 82201 Tel: 307–322–5553 Fax: 307–322–3283 Website: http://wdhfs.state.wy.us/ Media.aspx?mediaId=2281

Index

About the Author

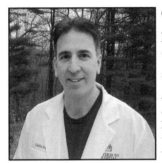

photo by G.S. Jayson

Charles Atkins, MD, is a board-certified psychiatrist working in Waterbury, Connecticut. He is on the clinical faculty at Yale University, and is the author of *The Bipolar Disorder Answer Book*. He has published five psychological thrillers and hundreds of articles and columns. His website is www.charlesatkins.com.